"Gary Marino has set off on what is sure to be one small step for man but one giant step for obesity!"

—*eDiets.com*

"Warning: Reading this book backwards could result in substantial weight gain!"

—*Comedian Tony V.*

"(It is) extraordinary…to go as public as Gary has gone to face a problem that has not been addressed previously in this way…"

—*Dr. Lee Kaplan—Massachusetts General Hospital Weight Loss Center*

"It takes a BIG man to realize he has a weight problem and Gary Marino is that man…well, not anymore!"

—*Jimmy Dunn—Comedian and TV Commentator*

"Gary has a powerful story to tell and anyone who has ever gone on a diet can relate to his struggles and challenges."

—*Todd G. Patkin, Dream Makers Charitable Endeavors*

"The best manuscript I've read at work."

—*On-Duty Clerk—Staples Copy Center*

Big & Tall Chronicles

Big & Tall Chronicles

✦

Misadventures of a Lifelong Food Addict!

Gary Michael Marino
Edited by Andrew Rechnitz

iUniverse Star
New York Lincoln Shanghai

Big & Tall Chronicles
Misadventures of a Lifelong Food Addict!

iUniverse Star
an iUniverse, Inc. imprint

iUniverse books may be ordered through booksellers or by contacting:

iUniverse
2021 Pine Lake Road, Suite 100
Lincoln, NE 68512
www.iuniverse.com
1-800-Authors (1-800-288-4677)

ISBN: 0-595-32154-2

Printed in the United States of America

This book is dedicated to the memory of my mother, Lorraine "Rainbow" Marino. You gave me the support and inspiration I needed to begin my road to health, and in turn I gave you everything I had on the road to The Million Calorie March.

October 2001

Contents

ACKNOWLEDGMENTS

Smart guy, that Ringo Starr. As far back as the 60s, he knew that surrounding himself with a little help from his friends was the best way to get through life. Of course if you are defeating a lifelong weight problem as I am, it may be a good idea to surround yourself with a lot of help from a whole lot of friends.

Many people contributed to helping me battle this disease, and their support directly influenced the material in this book. In the end, my body may have become smaller, but my heart has become larger, and it's because of these very special individuals.

I've often referred to the individuals directly involved in my health effort as my "Dream Team"—not because their work was particularly expensive, but rather due to the fact that they have helped this onetime hopeless food addict achieve his dreams—namely, to win control of my health and to help others. I'm forever grateful to my nutritionist Melinda Vaturro, R.D.; my therapist Ruth Schwartz, L.C.S.W.; my trainers Vincent Zarella, Sharon Cummings and the entire fitness staff at The Boston Sports Club in Lexington, Massachusetts.

Other professionals from Massachusetts General Hospital who provided additional support, education and expertise include Dr. Lee Kaplan of MGH's Weight Loss Program; Chief of Sports Medicine Dr. Bertram Zarins; and finally, my primary care physician, Dr. Jeffrey Harris.

My family's love and support is and always has been astounding. Love to my wife and Generation Excel Executive Director Julie Marino, my late mother Lorraine Marino, my father Leonard Marino, my late grandparents Ida and John LaCamera, Donna Marie Miller and her husband Tony, Laura Dean and her husband Leo, Richard Marino and his wife Josie, "Uncle" Dave LaCamera and his wife Karen, Alexandra, Mackenzie, Christopher, Brette, Devyn, Aunt Lee Mangiaratti, Michele LaCamera and her husband Douglas Maccaferri, my in-laws, Patricia and Bill Harmon and Linda and Ed Thorn, and finally my cousin, Andrew Rechnitz, for his amazing creative editing work on this book.

The inspiration for this book came from nearly three years planning "The Million Calorie March," the first cross-country walk for obesity. Friends who helped make that dream a reality include Matty Blake, Vinnie and Diane Sestito, Russell Surette, Brian Baldwin, Dan Jones, Dave McGillivray, Stephen Warshaw, June Knight, Denny Houghton Productions, Jim Gross and JRG Art, Leo Gozbekian Photography, Steven Richard Photography, Ellen Burnett, Linda Simon, Tony D'Amelio, Chris Zito, Ken Dicamillo and the The William Morris Agency, Boston City Councilor John Tobin, Representative Peter Koutoujian, Steve Grossman, Don Rodman, Bob Cotter and Ellen Gallo from Starwood Resorts, and finally the man who made the Florida to Boston walk a reality when all else failed: Todd Patkin and Todd G. Patkin "Dream Maker" Endeavors.

God bless Melissa Hurley, Wendy Mejia, Tricia Raynard and Rick Rendon at The Rendon Group, Boston and Jennifer and Adam Marko at The Marko Group, Jacksonville.

"A little help from my friends" also came from K.T. and Paul DiPanfilo, Honey Quigley, Bob and Nikki Garvin, Dr. Lillian Arleque, Susan Sloane, Norma Buckhaulter, Colleen Bleakney, Marco Discipio, Cheryl and Dave Slocum, Chuck and Mary Risch, John Cannava and Georgeanne Coleman.

Finally, I am deeply grateful to Boston comedians Tony V., Jimmy Dunn, Michael Coleman, John Turco, Tom Briscoe, Chris McGuire, Jon Stetson, Tom Hayes and Joe Yannetty for their creative input and contributions to this book. Laughter is truly the best medicine for overcoming any addiction. Thanks for writing the prescriptions, guys!

FOREWORD

I recently came up with a term to describe all the things in my life that I wanted but did not get. You may have heard of them referred to as "Broken Dreams" or "Unanswered Prayers" or even "Curses," but I now call them "Failure Miracles."

Like my childhood prayers that some day I'd play in the NBA. Each night when I went to bed my prayer was (from about ages 8-16), roughly translated:

"Now I lay me down to sleep—God please let me play in the NBA. I'll do anything. I'll be your humble servant boy on earth. I'll clothe the hungry! I'll feed the naked! Just please—me, NBA...do your thing!"

Guess what I don't do for a living?

Or things you don't want and get in bucketfuls. Like my pre-prom anxiety zits.

"God, please don't let me get zits before the prom."

Guess what happened as I lay in my bed the night before my prom? Pop! A big one right at the end of my nose. I could almost hear it come to life: *The zit heard round the world.*

As I grew older, my prayers and wishes became more serious. I begged harder and nothing seemed to come true.

I spent so much time cursing what I didn't have and lamenting what I did. What I wanted I didn't get. And what I got I didn't want.

It was only years later, looking back, that I realized these things were blessings. No, not just blessings, but miracles.

"God, why can't you give this to me?" eventually turns into "Thank God I didn't get *that!*"

Failure Miracles.

You would not be where you are today without them. As painful as they may be, they make you who you are. But here's the rub; you gotta make something of them.

Gary Marino has made something of his—big time.

Gary Marino, my friend and the author of this book, has known many successes, but he also had a really big Failure Miracle. He has endured a lifetime weight problem. He's addicted to something we all need: food.

How many times do you think Gary prayed,

"Please take this burden from me. Why can't I just eat normal? Like that guy? Why can't I just lose some weight and keep it off?"

I'm sure Gary would have killed for my little zit problem at the prom if it meant someone would take away a few pounds.

But nobody ever swept in and cured Gary. God never took away the food addiction. Gary struggled and lived the best he could, battling this problem for years, his prayers unanswered, or so it would seem.

See, if Gary had been born with a perfect physique, or if he had lost all the weight he wanted, every time he wished it, he would not be who he is. He would not have learned what he learned. He would not have become who he became—namely, one of the best people you could ever hope to meet.

What did he gain by having this weight problem? What did he gain having his prayers *unanswered*? Here's a short list:

- Mental toughness and inner fortitude.

- A beautiful and sharp sense of humor.

- Empathy for others.

- Patience in the face of real problems.

- Pride in the face of ridicule.

- Kindness in the face of the not-kind.

- Fierce determination with just the right mix of humility.

- Hope.

- And finally, it gave him a mission in life.

This book represents Gary's mission: to help others.

This book is the long-awaited yet blessed result of many Failure Miracles.

Gary lost this weight the hard way. No operations. No quick fixes. If you are looking for how a grapefruit can make everything okay, you've bought the wrong book. He looked inside, he made a stand, and he followed through. Now he shares all those things with you, using his journey to help you on yours.

So no, Gary never had his weight miraculously taken from him—thank God for that—for he would not be the person he is and so many people would not benefit from his awesome journey and inspiring story. So next time you don't get what you want, think "Failure Miracle." Think of Gary.

And thank whomever it is you believe in for their non-answer to your prayer.

Although…I'll still negotiate the NBA thing if you're listening, Big Guy.

And the zit thing was just uncalled for.

Matty Blake

PART I

PARADISE BY THE BUFFET LIGHTS

INTRODUCTION: GOING WIDE

Bourne, Massachusetts
July 1998, 11:35 pm

As I speed down Interstate 495 towards my uncle's beach house in Cape Cod, an eerie and familiar feeling returns to my mind and body. Behind the wheel, the white lines on the highway suddenly blur a bit through heavy, exhausted, almost hypnotized eyes. A warm, numb feeling slowly makes its way from the base of my spine up through the tips of my fingers. As a matter of protocol, I turn off the radio so I can concentrate on the impending problem. I open the window and moon roof to keep the wind in my face. In an instant, I am suddenly drained and paralyzed behind the wheel. I summon whatever little energy I can to keep my hands on the steering wheel. My foot seems permanently asleep as it applies pressure to the gas pedal. The car slows from 70 miles-per-hour to almost 50, but then begins to weave slowly in and out of the center lane. The cars in the lanes to the left and right begin to beep their horns and swerve defensively to avoid being hit by my four wheel death trap, which now seems in control of it's own destiny. I'm but a mere passenger in this horrific scenario, without even the energy to lift my foot off the gas pedal or turn the wheel to pull into the breakdown lane. Things suddenly begin to dim and my consciousness begins to fade. At 40 miles-per-hour, with cars in the lanes on both sides of me, my eyes begin to close and my head falls back against the headrest. I am not horrified or alarmed. This scene has repeated itself dozens and dozens of times for the past two years, and the only one truly responsible for this disease's powerful hold over me is myself. Although these episodes have become more and more frequent as of late, I am, for whatever reason, not afraid. The feelings of numbness gripping my body have lately become almost nostalgic in a sense, like an old friend I never asked for, like an old enemy I can't seem to get rid of. Long ago, I accepted these frequent losses of consciousness as my disease and became resigned to its hold over me. The scene has suddenly become quiet. I am in a deep subconscious state. By all rights, I should crash through the gates of Heaven any second. Suddenly a car horn plays loudly in my head. My brain goes from zero to 60 in half a second and my head snaps to the right in time to see the front of my car heading straight for the driver's side door of the car in the right hand lane. The driver is now leaning on his horn in hopes of avoiding the impending crash. Instinctively, with almost no input from my brain, my arms turn the wheel to the left with not a second to spare. Back safely in the center lane, I seem to be alert and in temporary control of my mind and body. Ahead, the Bourne Bridge takes me over the Cape Cod Canal, offering a breathtaking night view of Buzzards Bay and the quiet side of The Cape. At my uncle's beach house, family and friends are already fast asleep in anticipation of our usual weekend fishing and boating routine. They are, unfortunately, not the only ones fast asleep. On the other side of the bridge on Route 28 south, the white lines suddenly go blurry again. The scene I've just described repeats itself a few more times. With each episode I am amazed at how little warning I have. Once again the wave of exhaustion grips my body before I can pull over. As I drive towards Falmouth on a road that leads to the ocean, I suddenly slip into another coma-like state. At this late hour I am the only car on the road, but the road is a two-lane street that veers sharply to the left as it reaches the ocean. I am, of course, in no position to navigate a left. My head is back on the headrest and my eyes are closed. As usual, I have no control. Once again, everything is suddenly quiet. The silence itself is unnerving. Something deep inside my subconscious urges me to open my eyes and see what has become of my world.

I raise my heavy eyelids half-way. A white fence is heading for my car, or rather my car is heading for a white fence. I can make out the blackness of the Atlantic Ocean. In a second's time I spring into a state of complete alertness and slam on the brakes. The car skids loudly and stops only inches from the fence which blocks me from the rocky cliffs and dark waters below. My car stops, but my mind races with thoughts of how close I've just come to my demise. I can see the lights of Martha's Vineyard across the water, where by all rights I should be floating at this moment. I've come close before, but never this close. As I stare out at the ocean and digest what has just occurred, I can't help but ask myself how my life has come to this. Nearly two years earlier I had been diagnosed with sleep apnea, a disease caused, in my case, by weight gain and obesity. Can a man truly eat his way into a bizarre sleep disorder that threatens his very existence? The cold reality is that my life has come down to this. As a result, simple tasks such as driving have become nearly impossible. The tiny lights of the island are still shining at me from across the sea, creating a quiet, friendly haven in which to reflect on my mortality and begin the process of self analysis, perhaps for the first time in my life. I turn off the car's headlights, put my head on the wheel and ask myself where it all began...

Suddenly my mind goes back to a warm fall New England day in October, 1975. The orange, yellow and brown leaves were falling, literally raining down from the trees onto the Harrigan family's front lawn. My brother Rich and I, along with some neighborhood kids, were immersed in an intense game of tackle football. Mrs. Harrigan just happened to have the biggest front lawn on the street, and in those days, before we'd developed any real common sense, that was the only permission we needed to rip it up with our football antics. No need to ask. Have lawn, must play, you know?

"Go wide!" yelled the quarterback. Before I could look, the pass came to me from my left. As I jumped up and twisted my body to catch the ball, someone threw himself on me from the right and tumbled me to the ground. In typical neighborhood-game fashion, every kid pig-piled on me just to make sure I was "down." (Of course, before you feel bad for me, consider that I had been leading the pig pile just two plays before.) The last kid jumped up on the mountain of players on top of me. And that was when I heard it for the first time—the "F" word. No, not the four-letter word, but the three-letter one...F-A-T. Apparently someone thought I'd been gaining too much poundage and not enough yardage.

I slowly got to my feet and wore an awkward smile. I wasn't sure exactly how I was supposed to respond to an unsolicited insult of a personal nature. I waited for a referee to call him on an illegal use of the mouth, but the player who dropped the F-bomb continued his verbal pig pile. "You are. Look at you. You're fat," said the player who had unfortunately ended up underneath me when I was tackled. I kept a smile on my face, but felt embarrassed, and for the first time in my young life, extremely vulnerable. Meanwhile, the angry rant continued, while the game seemed to be on permanent hiatus. The other players stood in a circle, waiting to see how I'd respond. Apparently I'd taken the words "go wide!" too literally. I determined that this kid's anger was less about my impending weight problem and more about the fact that he had landed underneath me when he tackled me.

I figured it was a whole lot of 10-year-old 60-pound Italian landing on him at once. Nevertheless, the game went on without any further incident, and I used my new-found status as "the fat kid" to successfully tackle many players. Be that as it may, I'll never forget the first time someone publicly insulted my appearance. At age 10, I'd been introduced to the "cheap shot," and it had an impact on me. At that moment in my life, I was suddenly aware of my vulnerability to rude comments about my physical appearance. I wish it had been the last time, but it was only the first of many verbal and mental daggers to come that would assault my psyche and self confidence, essentially motivating me to eat even more to numb the anxiety.

Of course years later I did not take such insults as well. Cute little boys don't stay little or cute. They grow up to be hardened men who will defend themselves at any cost. It got ugly. Really ugly. But from that day on Mrs. Harrigan's lawn, I always felt that there was something deeply wrong with me. At a young age, my life had somehow become a left-hand turn and I seemed entirely powerless to stop it. My world had become like a movie that starts out great and then gets really stupid, and I'm sitting there in the theater with a Jacuzzi-sized popcorn (extra butter of course), saying to myself, "Do I really have to sit through this?" Don't get me wrong; I wasn't suicidal. I was just not up for watching this display of ridiculousness that my life was becoming due to my developing food addiction and weight gain. Psychologically, the disease had set me apart from other kids and I always felt one step behind everyone else. I was a person who needed to be fixed before he could move forward in life. Jobs, school, relationships, hobbies, careers—it all seemed to be affected.

Beyond my weight, I was always pretty different. I had Attention Deficit Disorder (ADD), and I was not much of an athlete so what chance did I ever have to be normal? My sense of humor, however, always helped me socially and kept me far from lonely. Eventually I learned that I was not alone in this struggle. In time I met others with the same food issues as myself.

Back on that day in 1975, however, I would never have believed that I and millions of other kids my age would struggle with our weight, damaging our health and enduring discrimination into our thirties. Never did think I would see a day when 65% of the country was overweight. One in three children born would develop type two diabetes and obesity that were linked to some fifty diseases, including the very deadly sleep apnea. And never did I think I would see the day when I'd become just one more statistic in some pediatric obesity file on some doctor's desk.

The kid's comment on the lawn that day, although innocent enough, sent me scrambling to learn about quick-fix diets and exercises, but it was already too late. The misadventures had begun.

GENERATION XL

"It came quickly, with little fanfare, and was out of control before the nation noticed. Obesity, diabetes and other diseases caused by diet and sedentary lifestyle now affect the health, happiness and vitality of millions…"

—*Dr. Kelly D. Brownell, PH.D.*
Director of the Yale Center for Eating and Weight Disorders

Looking back on it, my first Little League experience was probably an omen of things to come. On a chilly spring afternoon in the mid 1970s I was just another chubby, slightly freckle-faced kid signing up to play baseball in my hometown of Medford, Massachusetts. My folks, Leo and Lorraine "Rainbow" Marino sat shivering on the bleachers as 175 kids waited to be assigned to teams. It worked like some kind of junior draft system. Coaches scouted each kid at bat, on the bases and in the outfield. Depending on how a kid performed, he was assigned a team. If a kid was a good hitter but not much of a fielder, he balanced out the team in need of hitters. If a kid had all the right moves in the field, he was picked up by a team who needed solid defense. Me? I didn't really do anything right, but I had a good attitude and it worked. Other factors seemed to come into play as well. If a player was the son of a city councilor or lived on the same street as the coach, he stood a better chance of being picked by a talented team. Also, if a kid's young mother was known to attend games wearing a low-cut sweater or tight-fitting skirt, you could count on that kid being in demand as well. Medford, at that time, had some great teams. There were some great sponsors as well. Knox Photo had one of the best win/loss records around. Andre Realty had the best looking uniforms. Gaffey's Funeral Home wasn't the most inviting name for a baseball team, but they had one of the hardest throwing pitchers in the entire state. As the options dwindled down that afternoon, my time came and my name was called.

"Gary M. Marino," yelled the coach. "You're with McDonald's. Head on over." I remember my very first reaction. I thought, *McDonald's—Life is good!* The

Mickey D's Little League team had come in dead last the previous season, but I wasn't so much interested in the team's win/loss record as I was the much-talked-about incentive program I'd heard about.

"If you hit a triple," explained the coach, "you get a free Quarter Pounder with cheese. A home run gets you a free Big Mac". I remember thinking *And do I get fries with that? Hey, here's an idea. Why don't we drink strawberry shakes in the dugout instead of Gatorade. Why not chew Chicken McNuggets instead of chewing tobacco? On cold days, flaming hot apple pies could keep the players warm...*

The incentives on the McDonald's team were exciting, all right, but just in case that wasn't enough, every team victory was celebrated with a private party at—you guessed it—McDonald's. I didn't want to know what they offered as incentives over on the Gaffey's Funeral Home squad.

Every Saturday afternoon we put on our bogus blue and yellow McDonald's uniforms, which made us look about as intimidating as Ronald McDonald himself, and headed for the ball park to win some incentives. Now I couldn't hit a triple to save my life, but getting up at bat I was more fired up about the concept of the two all-beef patties and special sauce than I ever was about actually winning the game.

I guess I should have noticed my strong connection to food right then. It may sound like a cliché from a twelve-step program, but food truly was my friend. It was not fuel, it was love. Food had a kind of sixth-sense presence to me. It tasted beyond delicious. Food was what I lived for. It felt great going down and eating it always seemed to be front and center in my mind. Rather than list the foods I loved, I'll just make it easy and list the foods I didn't like: oysters, stuffed artichokes, fish cakes and liver. Have you got the picture? Everything else was fair game. Eating good food was pure rapture to me. I was drawn to it. I needed it. The powerful impulse to eat came from very deep within. From my earliest memory, I never seemed to have much control over it.

If ever a kid was truly cursed to grow up with a weight problem, I was still the luckiest cursed kid on the planet. Despite being at war with myself early on, I was born into an incredibly loving and nurturing family that remains close to this day.

Both of my folks were from working class, first-generation Italian-American families. Mom grew up in Cambridge, Massachusetts, and Dad on the streets of

Somerville. My sister Donna was the oldest, followed by my brother Rich, who was two years behind her. My little sister, Laura Jean, "the youngest one in curls," was two years my junior. Oh yeah, you guessed it—there I was, right there in the middle child slot. My problem, however, was not middle-child syndrome. Both my folks were masters at spreading the love into four equal parts. It was more like Chubby Midriff Syndrome.

Despite the troubles to come, I had good role models. Dad was a salesman and the proud family provider. Whatever we kids needed we usually got, as long as we approached Dad with Ma on our side. Ma needed no approaching. Her ability to tune into her kids and determine our individual needs was legendary. The quintessential mother of all mothers. Her nickname was born in Nantucket one year when a waitress asked her what her hippie name had been back in the 60s. "Rainbow," she responded. As the years went on, the name stuck because it was so fitting for a woman who radiated light and love. My dad, who usually went by the name Leo, had a nickname as well: "Labio". This nickname was coined by my mother in the late 80s after deciding he looked much like a bald version of the famous romance novel model Fabio. "Labio" was a great Italian cook who could be counted on each and every weekend to whip up amazing multi-layered lasagnas or massive antipastos with heapings of cheese, salami, eggs, and olives. You name it, it was in there. Rainbow was an even more outrageous cook. Her specialties were spaghetti sauce with meatballs, sausages, beef ribs and crown pork roasts with potatoes, onions, carrots and stuffing.

Between both parents, I was in a food funk pretty early on in life. My strong connection to eating continued to grow stronger as I got older. It was sheer addiction, combined with some solid Italian genealogy. The right to eat the foods I loved when I wanted was a big part of my very existence and I was always emotionally protective of that right. I was also acutely aware of my slowly building weight problem, but only half of me wanted to deal with it. The other half was just way too hooked on the concept of eating and it's soothing, tasty and instantly gratifying effects. Like most kids today, I probably watched too much TV when I should have been exercising.

My love of food was also compounded by environmental factors, such as the growing fast food industry. For myself and for an entire generation of kids, the 1970s were the test years for harmful marketing strategies such as "supersizing"—simply known as "large and extra large" back then—and merchandizing, with movie and toy tie-ins. The test was a success, and consequently it helped millions of children develop pediatric obesity in the years to come. What had been a "treat" in the 1950s and 60s had become a way of life for school-aged kids such as myself. The corporate giants were the only winners in this developing nightmare.

Eating shaped my childhood. However, it wasn't just the fast food industry that enhanced my love of food. Growing up in an Italian-American family was a front-row seat in the "Land Of Plenty." On holidays such as Thanksgiving and Easter, the festivities were not one day, but two. Aunts, uncles, grandparents, neighbors, therapists, family friends, household pets and anyone else with hunger pangs gathered around the dining room table, which was packed with mouthwatering dishes. The next day the same crowd reconvened around the table once again for the traditional leftovers. To not show up to the table on day two was the equivalent of being a "no show" on the holiday itself.

The next-day leftovers were an essential part of the holiday. I can still remember watching my Uncle David construct his glorious post-Thanksgiving Day "Turkey Gobbler Sandwich." First he would take a massive poppy seed roll, cut it in half and hollow out the dough with his hands, creating a sizeable crater. Then, with an entertaining look on his face that epitomized guilty pleasure, he would fill in the hole with mayonnaise, cranberry sauce and apple raisin stuffing. After piling on strips of white and dark turkey meat, he'd close the massive Dagwood sandwich, which now looked like an overstuffed suitcase, and put both hands on top, forcing the sides together. As he raised his Turkey Gobbler to his lips, I had to admit that it was a thing of beauty. One man's leftovers were truly another man's work of art. Later I noticed that I, too, had inherited this "artistic" ability.

Other traditions, such as the summertime cookout, became works of art as well. These ceremonies have been around since the pilgrims first broke bread with the Indians at Plymouth Plantation. By the time I was invited to the party, two hundred years later, the tradition of summertime cookouts were about putting yourself in a weekly kielbasa coma or deviled egg delirium.

Yet another tradition I loved was going to Boston's Fenway Park to watch the Red Sox play. Back in the mid-seventies, the team had a solid lineup and the pennant race was in full swing. For me, there were actually two races: The Pennant Race and the Concession Stand Race. The game was only half the attraction for me, much to my dad's dismay.

Petrocelli struck out? Bummer, can we go get a sausage?

Yastrzemski's up? Great, I feel like some kielbasa. Let me know how he does; I'm gonna get a Fenway Frank.

Bottom of the ninth with the bases loaded? Speaking of loaded, is anyone up for loaded potato skins? Can't be too many people in line at the concession stand. Indeed the score of the game, and whether my team won or lost, always seemed to be the sideshow. It was a good night as long as I was taking the full tour of the food vender stands.

My food addict antics never stopped. Each week I created traditions which only incorporated more calories into my lifestyle. On Sundays after church my friends and I split before communion to worship another holy deity: Brigham's banana splits. Before the church crowd even made their last sign of the cross, we'd be starting in on our ice cream sundaes. On the walks home from Mass, my friends and I hit the local convenience store for Chocolite Bars. Trust me folks, there was nothing *lite* in Chocolite Bars.

In fact, by the time I was a teenager there was nothing "lite" about me either. There is no doubt that food was overemphasized early on in my life. Like most Italian-American families, we celebrated food on a daily basis, "oohing" and "aahing" over every meal my folks put on the table. Of course once I developed my weight problem, food was celebrated one minute and taboo the next. The mixed message was confusing to an eleven-year-old. During the first serving, the family would talk about how good everything was. Then as soon as I reached for the second serving, suddenly it was bad to enjoy any more of it. A negative atmosphere came over the table, much like when an alcoholic reaches for another drink in front of his friends.

In the mid-seventies my family had settled into a perfect middle class neighborhood in West Medford, Massachusetts. It was full of kids and had all the innocence of The Brady Bunch. My older sister Donna was an honor roll student, competing in the Miss Massachusetts Pageant. My brother Rich was the high school's resident rock star with his band "The Legacy." My perky sister Laura was all straight A's and a cheerleader co-captain. Rainbow was a legendary angel, teaching crafts courses, running mother's clubs and rewriting the book on parenting. And Dad won the "Father Of The Year Award" in 1976. I was pretty much the only member of the family not pulling my weight. Actually that might have been the only area in which I succeeded. In hindsight, I didn't feel I was on the A-list of anything. I was just your average kid on a destructive path.

A BLOCK OFF THE
OLD CHIP

"Is that your dinner? I thought it was the centerpiece!"

—Leo Marino at the Cardoos Restaurant buffet

As I packed on the pounds, my sense of humor kicked proportionally into high gear.

"The family is so embarrassed about my weight problem they've hired the kid next door to play me in the family movies," I joked.

My ability to make people laugh primarily came from my mother and father. Dad had the ability to drop killer one-liners right smack in the middle of perfectly serious conversations. His brand of humor was upbeat and infectious. As a result, he was always the comic relief in social situations. Mom's humor was different, yet equally infectious. I guess a professional comedian today might describe it as "observational humor"—and her observations were absolutely hysterical. Rainbow could simply tell you a story about her encounter with a street performer during her lunch hour and have you rolling on the floor.

Sometimes my mother didn't even mean to be funny, but Rainbow always seemed to have a few "Mis-Adventures" of her own happening. By the time I was 11 or 12 it was apparent that I had inherited an equal share of both of my parents' personalities. Once my father realized that I'd developed a sense of humor, along with a weight problem, he quickly dubbed me "the block off the old chip."

My humor was a coping mechanism, of course. The truth was that I wished I had received some of my dad's other characteristics, such as athleticism, metabolism, work ethic and drive.

At any rate, sometime around August, 1976, Dad, perhaps noticing that the baby fat still hanging around his ten-year-old was a sign of trouble, signed my brother Rich and me up for Pop Warner Football.

"Do you guys want to play football this fall?" Rich and I exchanged equal "why not?" expressions and responded, "Sure Dad, great."

"I've already signed you both up," my father quickly followed up. "Tryouts are Monday afternoon and I've gone ahead and purchased some used pads and cleats." Rich and I looked at each other, realizing that Dad asking us about playing was more of an instruction than a question. I guessed we were playing football.

The field was littered with kids when we got to Playstead Park on that muggy afternoon in August. There had to be over 300 kids of all sizes milling about while their parents signed them up. It was a bit intimidating to see so many kids warming up. Not knowing where it all was going, I clung pretty close to my dad. Suddenly, a man in the middle of the crowd started yelling—not necessarily at me, just yelling abrasively in every direction.

"All right, line up! Everyone to the other side of the field!" the lunatic screamed. I clung even closer to my dad and looked at my brother to get his reaction. Why was this gorilla yelling? Had we done something wrong?

"Listen up and line up!," he yelled as he headed in our direction. "Everybody stop talking and line up at the other end of the field!" I looked up at my dad. *Should we leave?* Something had gone dramatically wrong, at least according to my 10-year-old brain. *This is already out of control. I agreed to play football, the same as we do on Mrs. Harrigan's lawn, only this time with nice big shoulder pads, cool uniforms and pretty cheerleaders. Maybe even a cool coach like Tom Landry from the Dallas Cowboys, who actually wears a hat and coat on the sidelines.* But there were no cheerleaders or cool outfits, and this guy was certainly no Tom Landry. This short hippie had shoulder length, dirty blond hair and an unshaven beard and mustache. He was wearing a tank top and gray sweats that barely fit his non-athletic, rotund body.

"You guys are gonna run!" he barked. "The longer it takes to get lined up, the longer you're gonna run!"

It wasn't even the look that was distressing. Hell, I'd been exposed to my share of hippies by the mid-seventies. It was the voice. That loud, angry, bullhorn voice. I'd never heard anything like it.

"Listen up! I'm not gonna say it again. Line up and get ready to run!" The man/beast walked over to where my brother and I were standing and pointed towards the far side of the field where the rest of the slain cattle were lining up. He barked, "Let's go! You guys get to the other side of the field and get ready to run! No one's doggin' it here!" My dad grinned down at me, almost as if to laugh at what a character this guy was. Assuming it was all some kind of joke, I left my dad's side and my brother and I headed to the lineup. It was there that I learned from the other kids that this coach had a nickname—"the Bulldog"—and it fit him like a collar. Eventually, with everyone on the line, the Bulldog looked in our direction and screamed, "I want sprints. One side to the other. No one stops until I say so!" This guy was mean. I thought, *where's the anger coming from, sir? We live in the suburbs, for Chrissakes.* The scene was all so over-the-top. I warily spied my dad all the way across the field. Now it was just parents watching and casually chit-chatting while their kids seemed to be sold into some sort of slave labor. I shot my brother an expression that said, W*hy would Dad sign us up for this?*

"Go, go, go, go! What are you guys waiting for!" screamed the Bulldog.

As we sprinted to the other side of the football field for the first time, I remember thinking it wasn't so bad, but this Bulldog kept screaming for more. And more. And more. And more. The pain in my body was more excruciating than anything I'd ever experienced in my life. My heart ached with each rapid fire beat. My calf and leg muscles burned as though someone had doused them with lighter fluid. There seemed to be no end in sight to this madness.

"You guys are still doggin' it!" Bulldog screamed. "We're gonna keep goin' until you stop doggin' it!" Already I was struggling to catch my breath. "Lets go! You guys are still doggin' it out there!" While I found it incredibly nauseating, the Bull Dog sure seemed to like the sound of his own voice. My brain was as shell-shocked as my body. I glared across the field angrily at my father. *Maybe* he'd *like to spend some time on the field with this animal.*

"All right, now, drop to the ground and give me sit-ups. No stopping until I say stop!" Sit-ups. Pushups. Leg lifts. Don't forget the jumping jacks and a side order of knee crunches. All of this with this Bulldog character screaming in my ear. All my brain could process was *When is this going to stop?* Out of the corner of my eye I continued to stare at my dad across the field, feeling that he'd betrayed me. He'd let this nut run me into a painful frenzy and just stood and watched. Where the hell was the football anyway? What about the part where I strategize, call the plays and forge ahead to the thrill of victory? The pain in my legs and stomach got increasingly worse. Just when I thought things would winding down, the Bulldog lined us up for something else. This time he had us sprint full speed in the direction of our parents. When we got two-thirds of the way across the field, at the sound of his voice (apparently a whistle was too quiet) we had to tumble on to our shoulders, roll completely back onto our feet, and continue running. *Run full speed at the ground. Great!* I thought. Of course by this time I was toast—mentally and physically shot. As I ran towards my dad, I looked at him as though he were a complete stranger to me. A sell out. I stopped, dropped and rolled, and for a minute I considered running into the woods. *Why bother?* I then thought, *It's almost over.* It wasn't over.

"All right, now I want everyone to run around the outside of the field ten times. And don't you let me see you guys doggin' it!" screamed the Bulldog. This guy's act was getting tiresome. Besides, who the hell was "doggin' it"? All I saw around me were kids coughing up tumbleweeds and running their butts off like me. As the final lap wound down, I began to strategize the revenge I would exact on my father for what he'd put me through. Maybe I'd never speak to him again. Maybe I'd go live with one of the neighbors. Maybe I'd find Ma a new husband. I wasn't quite sure, but I promised myself it would be brutal.

As I returned to the area where my dad was standing, I still hadn't made up my mind exactly how I'd handle the situation. One thing I knew for sure was that I would not make eye contact with the guy who had sold me out to this Bulldog animal, but as I approached him, our eyes mistakenly met. As sweaty and hurting as I was, the pain suddenly vanished. My dad smiled knowingly at me, almost as if to say that as crazy as it was, all of this was for my own good. I couldn't help but smile back, and I quickly forgave my father. In fact the excessive workout probably was for my own good.

As the weeks passed, the Bulldog seemed to lower his volume and lose his rabid edge. We learned he actually had a real name: Chuck…something. Much to our surprise, Chuck had a humorous side as well. When we were split up perma-nently into squads, Chuck seemed to be downgraded to league coordinator and I forged ahead to finish the football season as a solid second-string player. The point of my story is that even though I went on to play other sports such as base-ball, basketball, ice hockey, and lacrosse, I always associated exercise with great physical and mental pain. Perhaps that's where some of the initial trouble with athletics began. While the Bulldog may have simply been a character who loved playing with kids' psyches, my psyche has never been the same since that day in August, 1976. Never after that experience did I associate working out or getting in shape with anything but agonizing, unnecessary pain.

As a result, early on I decided to turn my attention to other things—like music. When I was 14, I bought a pair of used drums and convened my first rock and roll band, "The Boston Baked Beings." The name was a reference to the famous beans, as opposed to drugs. Even in our rehearsals, the food references never seemed to be very far away. "Okay guys," I'd tell my band, "let's rev up "Cheese Burger in Paradise" by Jimmy Buffet, then jump into "No Sugar Tonight" by the Guess Who. Tomorrow we'll learn a few tunes off of that new Meatloaf Album." A typical "Beings" set included tunes like "Ice Cream Man" by Van Halen, and down the line, "I want Candy" by Bow Wow Wow. I think you get picture.

In addition to music, I also developed other loves such as horseback riding. On Friday afternoons Rainbow would take me to the stables in West Medford where I would ride for an hour or more through the woods. My favorite horse? "Sugar-foot," of course. As I got older and more into horses, I began riding with a trainer. Eventually, as my weight ballooned, I backed off from horses altogether. Who wouldn't? Every animal has its breaking point, and I had no desire to see poor Sugarfoot go down into the mud like a mule.

Boating and tennis were two more hobbies that piqued my interest, but like horses, a chubby adolescent could only take those hobbies so far. Which brings me back to comedy and why, at an early age, I began to develop a sense of humor. Something told me I'd need one in order to survive with people like the Bulldog around.

Not long after the football season ended, my dad and I were building some wooden shelves at his workbench in the cellar. It was a Saturday, and we took a break from the job to have lunch. Dad made us both one and a half tuna sand-wiches on rye bread, with a lemonade for me and a beer for him. Dad finished his beer, but was still working on his sandwich when I had a glorious moment of inspiration. I grabbed his beer bottle, washed it out in the kitchen sink and filled it with cold water. I returned to the table just in time for my mom to walk into the room. With impeccable comic timing, I put the bottle to my mouth, aimed it straight up in the air and began gulping it down.

"Leo, you didn't give him a beer, did you?" Ma asked alarmingly. My father glanced across the table and couldn't have played along better.

"He's a man now, Lorraine," he responded, deadpan. Poor Ma. Here's her kid, already well on his way to a weight problem, and now someone's giving the 11-year-old a brewski.

"Leo, you didn't!" said Ma, becoming even more appalled.

"He's fine, he's worked hard today," my dad answered calmly. All the while, I continued to ignore them both and chugged the entire bottle. Dad watched, with a look of satisfaction on his face and nodded as though he were impressed by my ability to drink the entire beer without stopping. As the last of the water was drained, I wiped my mouth and slammed the bottle down like a good old-fashioned drunk. Rainbow, just short of a heart attack, realized that it was a joke and smiled at me adoringly. Later, I realized that that look was what life was all about.

"Ahhh, you're a block off the old chip, son," laughed my dad. That sense of humor, of course, got me through the many dark days when I was just a tormented kid, trying to understand his predicament.

The Art Of
THE ITALIAN
GRANDMOTHER

My grandmother Ida was born in Italy in 1911. She relocated to America in her teens and married my grandfather, John LaCamera, in 1931, just in time for the Great Depression. Notice the intoxicating combination occurring here? You've got a woman who's 100% Italian (meaning she's a killer cook who appreciates quality meals) immigrating to America and eventually living through a time when people rarely had enough food to eat or money in their pockets. Anyone who's ever known a relative who struggled during that time period in America knows the deal. The depression era folks were never the same again after experiencing such severe poverty. Everyone who survived it had a deep-seated fear of losing everything again. My grandmother had a basement you could only dream about. The family jokingly referred to it as "Ida's bomb shelter." Every type of food was neatly stored in cans and bottles, checked for freshness on a continual basis, and rotated accordingly. Pasta, tomato sauces, fruits, vegetables, candies (assorted types and flavors) and freezers stocked with fish, beef and chicken, all of which were neatly wrapped in wax paper and dated. While in high school in the early 1980s, we lived with the very real threat of nuclear war and I knew exactly where I was going should it ever actually occur: Gram's Bomb Shelter. "We'd be able to live for years down there," I used to tell my friends. "We'd probably die from clogged arteries if anything." I enjoyed a very close relationship with "Gram LaCam" right up until she passed away in 1992 at the ripe age of 81. Much of my childhood I spent with her and my mom. The three of us always seemed to be at some outlet store, bargain basement, or food warehouse. Years later, it occurred to me how sacred the shopping ritual probably was to a woman who lived through that depressing depression.

My mother's mother was incredibly sweet and loving, and yes, overweight since her twenties. She was funny and full of energy and at times right out of a television sitcom. Edith Bunker meets Estelle Getty meets Grandma Walton, the type of sweet, gray-haired old lady you could take to a biker bar and by the end of the night the Hell's Angels would be all seated around her on the floor, cross-legged and listening to her stories.

My grandparents were very much a part of my life growing up, which is just the way it should be. My brother and sisters and I all enjoyed the ritual known as the "sleepover." In true Italian Grandma tradition, food dominated the agenda, with all other activities penciled tentatively in between. True to Italian Grandmother tradition, food was love, and boy did Gram Lacam love us! In the morning you'd wake up to the smell of, well, almost everything. Gram's breakfasts were pretty damned amazing, considering she was cooking for one or two kids. Hot cereal, cold cereal, bacon, eggs, ham steak, sliced fruit, diced fruit, fresh fruit cups, assorted fruits, home fries, hot oatmeal, cold oatmeal…you get the picture. The table looked like an entire week's breakfast for the US Olympic Hockey Team.

Man, was it a beautiful sight! Gram was definitely into *abundance*.

As I grew older and acquired my driver's license, visiting her became a weekly ritual. When you grow up overweight, no one ever wants to feed you or see you eat. But with Gram, "No more, please!" meant *Just one more serving*. "Please, I can't eat another bite!" meant *Well, maybe one more serving if you feel strongly about it*. The woman lived to feed people, and the satisfaction and pleasure it gave her was evident in her beaming face. Walking in her kitchen door, Gram's opening line was always the same. "What can I get you?" she'd ask.

Gram's home was set up perfectly: You walked up the stairs to the side entrance of the house, opened the door and you were in the kitchen. Two feet to the right was the stove and the perpetual saucepot, which seemed to be glued to the front burner. It was always fired up, like the eternal flame. I used to wonder if the pot stayed put and the meats and sauces simply rotated. Ten inches to the left was the kitchen table, for easy access to the eating ritual. Twelve feet in front was Gram's refrigerator, standing proud in all it's glory. Just an arm's length away were all the supporting dishes—homegrown spices, and assorted cheeses for pasta—that you might need. No need to really get up. In typical Italian-Grandma tradition, she'd sit and talk to you and watch you eat. Everything Gram cooked had the distinct flavor of an old-fashioned, seasoned pro. The taste always amazed me. The woman could make a crown roast or something as simple as a grilled cheese sandwich and you'd think you were back in the old country. Even Gram's popcorn was popped, buttered and salted in a way that would make Orville Redenbacher consider another line of work. Gram's kitchen abilities were truly amazing.

"Gary, what can I get you?"

This was Gram LaCam's greeting before I was halfway through the door. What can I get you? What *didn't* she get me? Mouthwatering lasagna, penne pasta, broccoli chicken on ziti, spaghetti with meat balls and pork chops in red sauce, linguini with mussels and clams in white sauce, all prepared and seasoned to perfection. I have never experienced a cook like her to this day, and I consider myself a fairly well-traveled man.

Even when you weren't hungry, Gram's cooking could take you from zero to hungry in 5 seconds flat. A case in point was my grandmother's annual Fourth of July cookout at her home in Arlington, Massachusetts. At this blessed event, Gram always warmed up the crowd with her legendary honey and teriyaki chicken wings. They were broiled in a massive metal roasting pan and literally swimming in the delicious sauce. After bypassing the usual greetings with relatives, my brother and I hightailed it over to the roasting pan. Pop the cover. There goes one! Pop it again. That's two. Bang, a third, and a fourth, and a fifth. We're now heading towards six passes and I've not even yet greeted the bulk of my family.

As legendary as Gram's recipes were with the family, she had other talents, too. She could find nutritional value in just about anything. Pizza? "Well, the oil in pizza keeps your joints lubed," she'd explain, "and the vegetables on top of the cheese make up your entire daily allowance." Cheesecake? "Good for the whites of your eyes," she'd reason. Egg rolls? "Excellent for your ear canals." In hindsight, her philosophies were hysterical. "Finish that eggnog; you need the protein." God, I miss that woman! My grandmother also used adjectives that one normally wouldn't use to describe food. "Isn't that a handsome leg of lamb, Gary?" she'd marvel. "Aren't these veal cutlets I bought gorgeous?" Well, the woman was enthusiastic about her food, that was for sure. Gram had another great saying about pretty much any kind of food: It'll settle your stomach. "Have some hard candy; it'll settle your stomach." Ice cream? "It'll settle your stomach." Calzone? "Settles your stomach *and* holds you over till supper time."

But even an über-food lover like Gram Lacam had her limitations. I remember on one occasion, when I was sitting in her kitchen testing a couple softball-sized meatballs, I decided to book a flight to Florida for vacation. The airline's customer service line had many people on hold, including myself, so I decided to have a little fun with Gram. While on hold, I carried on a fake conversation.

"Flight 463?" I asked. "Sounds great. And what time does that board? Terrific. And do you know what the in-flight meal is? Chicken Cordon Bleu? Sounds good. And what do I get with this for sides?"

Grams eyes opened wide, as her incredulous expression changed with each passing second.

"Okay, what's the entrée served on the next flight?" I carried on. "Omelette? Okay. And how is that prepared? Can I special-order a ham and kielbasa? No? Well, are there any flights out the next day serving kielbasa with the meal?"

Right around this point Gram hit her breaking point.

"Gary, *abasta*!" (enough) she shouted.

Feeding people on airplanes was apparently over the top to Gram, but everything else was just fine. All was fair with love and food.

Gram even fed me in the hospital once, which wouldn't have been so crazy if she hadn't been the patient. It was winter, 1985, and Rainbow and I went into Boston's Brigham & Woman's Hospital to visit Gram after she had a back operation. As we walked through the door to her hospital room, Gram was righting herself to eat her standard hospital meal. "Gary, what can I get you?" my grandmother asked.

"Gram, you're in the hospital. You don't have to feed me," I responded.

"Well, just have the salad with a little bit of the chicken then," she pleaded. The sweet woman was actually feeding me some of her hospital meal. And did I partake? Well, what do you think? Anything for Gram Lacam.

The Late 70s:
LIVIN' LA VIDA LO-CAL

"It all starts innocently enough with a Milk Dud. Pretty soon you're looking for a bigger kick, like a Mounds. Now you're in the life—popping truffles, sharing pixie sticks. Then one day they find you in an alley, mainlining Jujubes."

—*WB Network Pilot*

Halloween 1977. As the chubby ringleader of our neighborhood gang, the 'Cardiac Kids,' I began hatching a plan to maximize our candy intake that year.

Looking in the rearview mirror, I'd always handled my Halloween candy differently from my siblings. In the late 60s and early 70s, it was always about evading my father. It wasn't that he cared that I was overdosing on candy like every other kid on Halloween. It was that he wanted in on the action. Dad was a guy with a sweet tooth, and our trick or treating was to his benefit. The tradition was innocent enough and it was pretty much the same every year. Rainbow hooked up with the other neighborhood moms and took us kids out door-to-door. When we returned home, my dad would be watching TV in his traditional 1970s Archie Bunker low-rider. "All right, guys, flip your bags over on the floor. I really should test this stuff before you eat it," Dad would say with his trademark sarcastic smile. And there we'd all be, sitting on the floor around Dad's easy chair, watching with nervous smiles as he brushed through the piles of Hershey Bars, Milk Duds, Butter Fingers, licorice sticks, and M&M's. Usually it would be my brother Richie and myself with the biggest piles, and the girls sitting next to us with slightly smaller ones. All of us wore tortured looks at the thought of losing some of our hard-earned Halloween stash. Dad would pick a few things from each of our piles and form his own pile on his lap. As soon as he turned his attention back to the TV, we seized the opportunity to scoop everything up as fast as we could, back into our bags. We stashed them in our rooms, under our beds, or wherever they'd be safe, not just from our father, but from each other. The tradition of nightly inspections by my father continued for about two weeks, until eventually the candy was whittled down to the usual melted Reese's Peanut Butter Cup. You know, the one with the wrinkled and worn plastic wrapper.

By the time I was 11 or so I had developed a solid plan to keep the candy around clear through the Christmas season. As soon as we returned home from trick-or-treating, I headed for my room, where I split my candy windfall into a second bag: a decoy bag, if you will. Most of the second string candy (stuff I could live without) went into the decoy bag: caramels, candy corn, apples, Necco wafers, sour balls, and the like. The entire island of misfit treats were collected in the decoy bag. Then I'd head downstairs with the impostor bag to let Dad go through his "testing" ritual. There I'd be, sitting next to my sisters and brother, legs folded, grinning up at my father and letting him purge my Halloween stash to his heart's content. Nobody ever seemed to question how incredibly weak my candy take was, or the fact that weeks later, when everyone else's candy was long gone, I'd spend quality time with Milky Ways, Snickers Bars and Oh Henrys. In other words, the royalty of the chocolate world. Oh yeah, little Gary was a hold-out, but I had even better shenanigans just waiting to be hatched.

By 1977 it was clear that I was on my way to at least a marginal weight problem. However, undaunted and in full adolescent denial, I forged ahead. One of my first friendships was with a *young rebel without a cause* type named Kelly Michaels. In many ways, Kel and I were typical kids. We played sports with the other kids from the neighborhood and we caused trouble whenever we could get away with it. We had our rooftop hangout, called 'the Skyline,' located conveniently on top of my neighbor's garage. The Skyline was littered with *Playboy* magazines heisted from somebody's trash. Miss April was hanging proudly from the tree branch that kept the entrance to the Skyline hidden. Miss August, Miss February and Miss December also hung from the branches. As a result, the Skyline didn't have much of a view of the sky at all, but in our minds it was the top of the world.

At any rate, by Halloween we had assembled a group of kids from our block who were young, crazy, and willing to go along with our antics for all the wrong reasons. A new twist to the trick-or-treat tradition had been discovered around this time, none other than the art of egging and shave-creaming. Kelly's specialty was spraying the foamy shaving cream on household pets that were sitting on the front stairs of the homes we visited. Mine was throwing eggs at teenager's cars as they drove by, especially the ones acting way too cool. Pre-teen adolescence was in full bloom. But as fun and innocent as these traditions were, Kelly and I were not exactly ready to let go of the best part: the Halloween candy.

By October 31st we had come up with a scheme to accumulate a little—okay, a lot of extra candy. Kel and I built a life-sized scarecrow using leaves and some old clothes. For the head we bought a full-length, three-dimensional Frankenstein mask and fastened it onto the scarecrow's body. An old pair of rubber boots with iron rods duct taped to them served as Frank's feet. Once fastened correctly, the dummy could not only stand on it's own, but from a distance looked pretty life-like, or at least enough like a trick-or-treater who could collect candy for a couple of wise guys like us. The problem was that the hands were a dead giveaway. Of course the fact that the dummy couldn't talk didn't help either.

"What if we tie his hands to a trick-or-treat bag and leave him in the shadows on the sidewalk?" I asked.

"That'll work!" replied Kelly.

Cut to nighttime on the 31st. The streets are full of trick-or-treaters going door to door. Two 12-year-olds dressed as winos are taking their "kid brother" around to neighborhoods all over town. "Could we also get some candy for our brother Frank?" we'd say as we motioned to the dark figure watching from under a tree. "He's a little shy."

In the shadows, Frank would be standing with trick-or-treat bag in hand. By the end of the night we were back at the Skyline, dividing up the dummy's treat bag while Frank lay abandoned in three pieces twelve feet away. All things considered, our shenanigans were innocent by today's standards. But life does have a way of catching up to you, doesn't it?

By the spring of 1978 I was wearing my love for food on the outside and my mom, knowing all too well what my life would be like with a weight problem, began putting a plan into place.

The basement of Medford's Fowler Dance Studios housed the local chapter of Weight Watchers International. The group met once a week on Wednesday or Thursday evenings and Ma seized the opportunity to get me involved in a healthier lifestyle.

"You know I love you no matter what you weigh," she'd say.

There it was, the official introduction to every subsequent conversation concerning my weight problem. Mom was always aware that broaching the subject of my looks could negatively effect my self-confidence. I was, after all, a twelve-year-old boy trying to develop a little self-esteem, so Ma made sure I would not go alone. Her friend Elena had a son who was in a similar predicament—young, active, "husky" and clearly on his way to a life-long weight problem. Michael was a nice kid who attended the same Catholic grammar school as I did. While we were aware of our parents' friendship, we had never been particularly tight. Beyond seeing each other at St. Joseph's School, our relationship had been limited to the occasional basketball competition or backyard game of catch whenever our mothers got together to chat and have tea. In the spring of 1978, however, Mike and I were about to bond on a much deeper level. Well, as deep as thirteen-year-olds get.

"Elena is bringing her son Michael to Weight Watchers," my mom said. "He's joining the program, so you two can do it together!" *That's great Ma, and will some of the nuns from St. Joseph's be joining us as well?* I remember thinking sarcastically. The young rebel in me wanted to reject the offer to go, but in hindsight, it may not exactly have been an offer at all. More like an order. Regardless, something deep inside told me that joining Weight Watchers might be in my best interest, especially with the high school years looming just around the corner. So on a warm night in May the four of us made our way to the basement of the dance studio. A typical scene for 13-year-olds it was not.

As we made our way down into the bowels of the building, we encountered a major distraction. Young dancers were spread out everywhere, coming and going from dance classes on the main level. "What a country!" I joked to Mike. "We've been here 5 minutes and already I'm inspired!" I quipped. Our enthusiasm would not last long. Continuing down the stairs and into the sweaty, humid, cramped room where the Weight Watchers group met, Mike and I noticed the dancers were now virtually extinct. Replacing them were 40 or so middle-aged women who were clearly in the midst of their own weight loss struggles. We couldn't have been more out-of-place. Mike and I did our initial weigh-ins and then took our seats for the nightly lecture. "I'm so-and-so, I've lost 35 pounds, I've kept it off for more than 6 years and I'm excited!" was the battle cry. Three hours earlier I'd been watching Moe, Larry and Curly, and now I was supposed to bond with Maureen, Lorna and Cathy. It just didn't grab me. Well, not at first, anyway.

Rainbow and I decided that although the Weight Watchers program gave the dieter plenty of food options, my best shot to lose weight was to design a daily and weekly food plan, utilizing the guidelines from Weight Watchers International. The plan that would serve as my eating bible would be pinned up on the refrigerator door, just in case I needed to check to see if ice cream sandwiches were allowed or not. The plan was healthy, but not exactly ground-breaking. Hard-boiled eggs where cereal had been. Sliced turkey breast where Italian cold cuts had been. Salads where nothing had been. The wonderful invention known as "the rice cake" had not been discovered yet, thank God. Skim milk, fruit, or yogurt as a mid-morning snack. It was essentially a *spin-off diet*. If the Weight Watchers plan was a sitcom like "All In The Family," my diet was more like "Archie Bunker's Place." The winning ingredient of the plan Ma and I designed was not only what foods I was eating, but having them assigned every day in advance. In hindsight, it was probably the only way a kid with ADD could follow a diet. I'd wake up in the morning and head for the diet plan taped to the refrigerator. In typical food-lover fashion, I'd eat my breakfast while reading what was in store for lunch.

By the second week's weigh-in, Mike and I were feeling the low cal love. Mike came out of the gate with a quick 3 or 4 pound weight loss. I quickly followed with 2 or 3. Then we took our seats for the weekly "I'm so-and-so, I've lost 35 pounds, I've kept it off for more than 6 years and I'm excited!"

Around the third week of Weight Watchers, my other grandmother, Nana Marino, came up from Florida to stay with us as she did every year at that time. Unlike Gram LaCamera, "Nana Marino" was blessed with a good metabolism and exercise ethic. So at 4 foot 11 inches, she was in phenomenal shape. Nana Marino noticed the Weight Watcher's diet hanging on the refrigerator that summer and made me an offer I couldn't refuse. She said, "I'lla paya youa tennadollars pera pounda youa losa!" (that was ten American dollars per pound for those of you not skilled at interpreting Italian-style broken English). I quickly added it up, figuring I had at least 20 pounds to lose. I remember thinking *Wow, over $200! That's more money than I've ever known. Being fat can really pay off!* By the third week of Weight Watchers, Mike and I had put up a solid weight loss of fifteen pounds between the two of us, but the motivational rap at every meeting had begun to get old. "I'm so-and-so, I've lost 35 pounds, I've kept it off for more than 6 years and I'm excited!" By this time Mike and I had developed a plan. We'd leave our moms (who went with us religiously every week) and head upstairs to gawk at the dancers from the rehearsal studio under the guise of "Let's go get a Tab." Tab was the world's first diet soft drink. To me it tasted simply awful, but it had zero calories and was the standard-issue beverage for folks like me who were involved in the battle of the bulge. The dancers always seemed to overflow into the hallways and dressing rooms. "No need to hear any weight-loss stories downstairs, Mike," I'd joke. "All the incentive we'll ever need is right up here." By this time Mike and I were like blood brothers, chasing girls and playing badminton in his back yard for hours at a time. We never talked about Weight Watchers, not publicly and not to each other. You would never catch us polishing off our lunches at school asking one another about the amount of calories in a pint of strawberry milk. It was like the Junior Knights of the Round Table, a secret club we belonged to. By day we were typical schoolboys, but by night we knew we'd be seeing each other in the basement of the dance studio. It was bizarre, to say the least.

At any rate, by the late summer of 1978 both Mike and I were looking trim and fit. *Hi, we're Gary and Mike, we've lost 40 pounds between us and we'd like to thank our mothers and the dancers upstairs...*

The Weight Watchers diet plan had worked. By the fall of that year I'd lost twenty pounds and my chubby stomach and love handles were gone. Rainbow was ecstatic as she reached for the camera on that first day back to school. "Smile!" she gushed. The dream had been realized. Later, when I scrutinized the photo, I had to admit that I really did look different. And as for that $10 per pound incentive plan? Well, by the following spring sweet Nana Marino, 75 or so at the time, had begun to lose her memory a bit. She remained a chatterbox for many more years until her death at 90, but the incentive deal—or anything else in recent history—seemed to be lost to her. Don't think for a second I didn't try to jog her memory.

"Nana, remember me?" I'd plead. "$10 per pound? What do you say we go a buck a pound. Hello? Nana?"

Despite my newfound fit and healthy look, returning to school that September put me back into the same junk food eating circles I'd left in June. In fairly short order the program at the dance studio began to look like just another summer camp-like experience to me. At 10:30 every morning my schoolmates and I would buy 2 bags of potato chips from the "Chip girl" who dipped by our classroom. They were fifteen cents per bag. The chip sales raised money for the school and were intended to be eaten with lunch, but eating them while the teacher's back was turned was a daily guilty pleasure. As a result, we quickly became experts at keeping our crunching down to an inaudible level. At lunch we'd swipe extra pints of chocolate milk from the cafeteria refrigerator to augment our peanut butter and fluff sandwiches. You can see where this is going, can't you? A couple times per week the nuns would pick two students to take the bank deposits to downtown Medford Square. This was a score on two levels. First, we'd take extra long to get the job done so we'd miss class. Secondly, we'd stop by the local ice cream parlor or a donut shop and feed our faces to our heart's content. Whatever the reasons had been for attending Weight Watchers were quickly forgotten. My old friend "Food" was back, and I welcomed him with open arms. Old traditions returned. I'd gather all of the Crunch Berries from Capt'n Crunch Cereal and have myself a bowl of straight sugar when nobody else was watching. Then I'd snort the Crunch Berry dust and hit the freezer. Slowly and methodically I would unravel the tape and string from the boxes of Rainbow's frozen cookies or brownies, quickly pop four in my mouth and then spend hours putting things back so my break-in would go undetected.

If only then I'd known the damage I'd be doing to my metabolism by losing and gaining weight, maybe I'd have taken a second to think about the eventual impact of things. But at the age of 14, I'd lost the will to go back to depriving myself of the foods I loved.

By the beginning of 1979, the twenty pound weight loss and entire episode were all history. The Weight Watchers plan still hung on the refrigerator, but by now it was wrinkled, faded, and almost invisible to me. Now, in my final months at St. Joseph's School, daily life included lots of TV and whatever was in the kitchen cabinets that I could put a hit on.

At night, mainly on weekends, I'd begun experimenting with beer drinking and partying. The experiment was a success! I was able to drink nearly a six pack and a half by my 15th birthday. For my friend Mikey, the scenario was very different. Mike kept the weight off, stayed active and looked great. I was always looking to see if Mike would gain his weight back as well. But by and large—or not so large—Mike was as trim and fit as he was after that summer of 1978. How he did it was always a mystery to me. Nevertheless, I'd always hear it from members of my family. "I ran into Mike today. He looks terrific! He's kept the weight off." As nice as Mike was, I began to develop a deep-seated resentment toward him. He'd succeeded where I'd failed, and everybody seemed to take note of it.

As the years went by, I occasionally bumped into Mike on the bus or at a family get-together and he was as gracious and friendly as ever. He always invited me to hook up, but I ended up putting a wall between us. It seemed to me that Mike had forged on to live a normal life and do all of the things I wanted to do, but I was stuck. His very existence reminded me of my failure and of my mom's disappointment. The kid had done nothing to me, but I always steered clear of any genuine relationship. I don't think he ever figured out why.

Not terribly long ago I ran into Mike, his wife, and his son Michael Jr. on Cape Cod. He was fit, healthy, good-looking and maintained the same optimistic personality he possessed during our junior high school days together. He asked if I was interested in coming to an annual fall get-together with some friends at his home. I politely declined.

BIG AND TALL CHRONICLES

"Fat, drunk and stupid is no way to go through life, son."

—*Dean Wormer, National Lampoon's "Animal House" (1978)*

The blue beam of light from the flashlight made its way from the license plate over to the "Medford Lacrosse" bumper sticker, and then slowly up the side of the brown 1972 Ford Torino. The light then flashed towards the front seat, where the low, guttural moans were coming from. The two individuals inside had adjusted their seats to the recline position, leaving them completely unaware of the policeman's light shining through the back seat and onto the backs of their headrests. In the moonlight, a male voice blurted out "Oh my God, is that good!" More moaning followed. The officer smiled for a second and considered leaving the young couple, clearly high school kids, to experience life's pleasures without interruption. This was the Mystic Lakes region of Medford, Massachusetts, and had been a lover's lane for many years. Just a few short years ago, the officer himself had probably parked there to experiment with his high school sweetheart. As the officer turned to leave, a second male voice—this one lower—announced, "Are these ribs hittin' the palatal G-spot or what?" The officer suddenly flung the driver's-side door open with disgust. The two high school boys looked up, only half distracted from their foil-lined platters.

"All right, both of you out of the car!" he commanded. "Wipe those stupid smiles, and while you're at it, that barbeque sauce, off your faces, and explain exactly what the hell is going on here!"

What in fact was going on were two school kids spending more quality time with ribs than anything else. For me, it would not be the last time. My restaurant career was just beginning.

My first job in the industry began in the fall of 1979 at a quiet Chinese restaurant along the banks of the now-famous Mystic River. The Bean Villa was a modest-sized restaurant, with an even more modest following. It had opened up just a few years earlier to less than spectacular reviews. From that time on, with the exception of a table here and a table there, things were pretty sleepy. However, all of that was about to change in late 1979. That was the year that Joseph Spinazzola, the premiere food critic in Boston (the Annual Spinazzola Benefit, held in his memory, is today one of Boston's biggest food events), wrote a stunning A+ review about the Bean Villa in the Boston Globe.

After the word got out about the food, the place went from decaf to speed-ball—an overnight sensation—at least until the brothers Marino and friends arrived on the scene, after which the rating would take more than a slight dip, to roughly a D-. But don't let me get ahead of myself.

When the rave review came out, the Bean Villa was clearly caught off guard. The figure I remember hearing was that 150-250 people were being turned away per night. The restaurant was in trouble and was badly hurting for waiters, kitchen help, dishwashers, and anyone who could service the masses. So as fate would have it, in late 1979, my mom was sitting in a friend's hair salon next door to the restaurant when its exhausted managers came in to inquire with the salon's owners about getting some bodies to help out. Ma's ears perked up, always looking out for her boys, and within twenty-four hours my brother Rich and I had jobs. The owners not only offered great hourly pay, but more importantly, the chance to order anything you wanted to eat off the menu at the end of every night. It was an exciting offer, and I was grateful. However, this chubby Italian kid was hardly waiting for the end of the night to eat. An hour into my first shift I'd already constructed a methodology to enjoy the perks of working in a tasty Chinese restaurant. First I developed and fine-tuned the 'Clip Method.' Here's how it worked. When the Chinese waiters walked up the stairs from the kitchen with fresh platters of food, I keenly took notice of the peculiar angles at which they held their trays, basically resting them on their shoulders and balancing them behind with one hand. The key word here being *behind*. There would be a moment, a half second at most, when they would walk through the swinging doors from the back room where I worked into the main dining room. If my timing was right, the tray with the food would still technically be in the back room, but the waiter would have already passed through the doorway. This was the moment to make my move. With magician-like sleight of hand I would reach up and grab a spare rib or a chicken finger and scoff it right down. Here today, gone in a second. An egg roll here, pork strips there, and the occasional teriyaki stick (these were easier to clip off the waiter's platters because the wooden sticks hung way off the trays). To my amazement, no one ever seemed to notice that the heisted items were missing from the Pu Pu platters or dinner entrees. When my brother Rich and our friends began to notice how successful my clip method was, they began using it as well. By the end of the night I never seemed to be hungry, but that never stopped me from taking the owner's offer to order anything we wanted off the menu.

"Anything" meant everything. Hello Pork Fried Rice, Beef Lo Mein, Chicken Wings, Crab Rangoon and anything else that seemed even mildly appealing. In hindsight, I should have noticed then where the line of reckless teenage eating stopped and a problematic food addiction began. It was tough to see amongst the chaos created every night in the Bean Villa's back room. That's because hiring me was not the only mistake the owners of the restaurant made back then. The other was inviting Richie and me to, as they put it, "hire any of your friends who are looking for jobs." In no time the Bean Villa was overrun with teenage boys and pandemonium quickly ensued. Drinking on the job, ferocious water fights, new clip methods, dumbwaiter rides, and general "Animal House" type madness. I wouldn't have batted an eye if John Belushi himself had walked through the door in his famous Samurai getup.

I was quickly demoted from waiter to dishwasher after pouring cold water down a young woman's blouse when she asked for a refill. No big deal. As head dishwasher, I not only excelled at the water fights by using my power nozzle on the wait staff, but I also worked dangerously close to the freezer, where the fried ice cream was kept. This was a Bean Villa special dessert, and a delicious one at that. Deep-fried vanilla ice cream the size of a softball, with a coating like Rice Krispies. Mighty good. From my dishwashing station I could walk around a corner, grab 4 or 5 out of the freezer, and make a beeline for the back door, which brought me out to the darkness on the banks of the Mystic River. Of course I always bumped into a few of my friends out there. They were up to no good, drinking beer that was "borrowed" from the bar, or eating the contents of some poor guy's hijacked Pu Pu Platter. The fried ice cream didn't last very long outside in the night air, so our standard procedure was to take a couple of bites and pitch the dessert right into the river. Below the waterline, I could only imagine the Wonder Bread-eating fish gnawing on those for weeks.

Between my sudden 30-pound weight gain and weekly almost-firings, business at the restaurant, not surprisingly, began to fall off. The boys and I were no longer needed, most likely thanks to our own antics. With us gone, life soon returned to normal at the Bean Villa. As much as we missed the "anything you want off the menu" routine, we were young, full of energy and ready for new adventures.

By 1980 I was just another chubby freshman at Medford High School. Between my failed Weight Watchers diet the previous year and my Bean Villa antics, I was becoming very self-conscious about my size. By this point, the taboo of being overweight had been thoroughly drilled into my head. At that time, I understood that my life would be a left-hand turn unless I got thin. I was also beyond the cuddly schoolboy age, and talking about weight with people was entirely off-limits. I didn't want to hear about it from Rainbow, my family, or my school mates, even though these conversations were never far away.

By the spring I'd taken matters into my own hands with my very first attempt at a starvation diet. As far as I was concerned, I'd already tried it their way by carefully measuring foods, counting calories and posting my daily regimen up on the refrigerator. Now I was going to try it my way. I proceeded to go entire days without eating one thing—no breakfast, lunch or dinner. I decided if I couldn't have it all, then I wanted none of it. The future was coming and there were parties to frequent, cheerleaders to date, and sports championships to win. Oh, the glory I had in mind for myself! During these desperate starvation diets, I somehow managed to live on water with the occasional glass of orange juice. Brilliant, huh? By the fourth day, as you can imagine, I would crack under the pressure. Usually I would be in the school cafeteria, with every intention of just socializing. Then my buddy Dipa would walk in. His family owned DiPasquales' Italian Restaurant in South Medford. South Medford was sort of our version of Little Italy. Dipa's family would hand-craft a beautiful Italian cold-cut sandwich on fresh bread every day and send it to school with him for lunch: sliced salami, fresh mortadella, and imported Italian prosciutto. They were all present and accounted for and I can still remember the sight of the oil and vinegar dripping out as he unwrapped that baby on the table in all its glory. "Gorgeous," Grandma LaCamera would have said. My friends and I enviously watched as he lifted the enormous grinder to his lips. Oh, the humanity! But as the old saying goes, if you eat filet mignon everyday, it starts to taste like hamburger. The attraction apparently began to wear off for young Dipa by the spring. That's when he offered me his massive sandwich in exchange for lunch money. I reached for it like a guy trapped in the desert without water. So long, starvation diet. Hello, assorted Italian cold cuts! Even if Dipa wasn't around, three or four days without proper nutrition would make anything look utterly tempting. Once I made up my mind that I couldn't take it anymore, I usually headed straight to the cafeteria for ribs, corn on the cob, some kind of a petrified chicken thing and mashed potatoes that could grout bathroom tile. Despite the standard issue cafeteria food, hamburger suddenly began to taste like filet mignon. Inevitably, I paid the price for my starvation outings, and by the beginning of my sophomore year had gained everything I'd lost—plus more. I knew nothing at this young time in my life about damaging the body's metabolism, lowering metabolic rates, or the stress put on the body due to rapid weight gain. I only knew how to eat more and more, which made me happier and happier. And how fitting that in 1981 a new restaurant called "The Happy Haddock" had become all the rage in town.

The Happy Haddock was serving up fresh seafood, BBQ steak tips & chicken wings in a new revolutionary sweet-style marinade. The restaurant was owned and operated by Anthony Ruggieri Sr. and his two sons, John and Anthony Jr. Rumor had it that they had paid big money for the exclusive rights to the magic marinade recipe. I quickly understood why: *it was worth it.* The marinade was a delicious blend of Ah So sauce, brown sugar, honey, corn syrup, and sparerib glaze. Okay, I'm speculating here. Honestly, I don't know to this day what was in their prized marinade. It was always shrouded in secrecy. All I knew back in '81 was that the owners guarded the recipe with their lives and I was addicted to the tasty red marinade from the minute I met it. The restaurant opened in 1980 and was an immediate hit. The Ruggieri brothers were young, restaurant-savvy and excited about their new establishment. They had something else they were pretty excited about at the time, too—a stellar new employee named Richard Marino. My grandfather, John "Jiggsy" LaCamera, had honed my brother's work ethic and stamina just a few years earlier, working maintenance at a nearby shopping mall after the Bean Villa gig dried up. My grandfather picked him up at five in the morning and worked the kid to the bone. In the process, however, he instilled some hard-working habits in my brother that continue to this day.

The Ruggieri family raved about my brother and reveled in the idea of recruiting his younger brother as well. After all, two Richie Marinos? How much better could it possibly get? Looking back, of course, what a disappointment they'd set themselves up for. Within two weeks I'd reassembled my crew from the Chinese restaurant. A typical day for me at the Happy Haddock went something like this. I'd drink alcohol with my co-workers in the parking lot before our shift, and then eat a half dozen or so fresh rolls in the dressing room while getting ready for work. Then I'd "test" all the fresh onion rings and steak tips for quality-control purposes. At break time I would order a half-priced entrée. Finally, towards the end of the night, we'd make arrangements with the kitchen crew to acquire more beer for the next day's shift. In many ways I'd simply resurfaced my Bean Villa gig at the steak and seafood place up the street. One day my brother approached me with a sheet pan of hot Ruggieri's ribs and asked me to cut the racks into individual ribs for the dinner crowd. After doing that, I invited my friends, who were now part-time employees as well, to sample the product line. By the end there were two measly orders of ribs at best. My brother smiled and shook his head. "Little brother's at it again," said Rich. My brother always had a sense of humor about my work ethic, or lack thereof. His reputation as a strong, hard and incredibly fast worker stayed intact, despite my shenanigans.

By late summer I was convinced that only one thing could be better than Ruggieri's tasty marinade: Ruggieri's tasty marinade at home several nights per week. I envisioned homemade buckets of the stuff in my mother's refrigerator at all times. *That would be the ultimate,* I thought to myself. But how could I reproduce it on my own without knowing the ingredients? I decided to ask the owners one last time, but once again they politely brushed my request aside. They were wholesome, hard-working brothers, not unlike my brother Richie. I was cut from a different cloth, however, and once again the fix was in.

I conspired to take a sample of the stuff home to our kitchen, study its ingredients and reproduce it on my own. Pretty enterprising for a kid, eh? One hot Saturday, as my shift was winding down, I slipped into the giant walk-in refrigerator where the barrels of marinade were stored. I pulled a ladle from my sleeve and a plastic sandwich bag from my pocket and quickly scooped a generous amount of the blood red marinade into the bag. I tied the top of the bag and slipped it under my white work shirt, just below my rib cage. The problem was that these were the days before Ziplock bags. As I sat outside the restaurant on a curbstone, waiting for Rainbow to pick me up, the bag burst beneath my shirt. When Ma pulled up in her shiny blue 1979 Toyota Corolla, I approached the car with a massive blood-colored stain around my midriff. I saw a look of horror come over Rainbow's face. There was her sixteen-year-old, holding a stomach full of blood. I walked over to the driver's side window to assure her I'd not been machine-gunned. When I explained the story of the marinade to Ma, that look of unconditional love and adoration came over her face again. She may not have been crazy about my antics, but I could do no wrong in her eyes. It became one of her favorite stories for years.

Eventually, I began to realize that it was only a matter of time until the nice folks at the Happy Haddock caught on to my shenanigans and showed me the door, so in November of 1981, I abruptly quit. The owners weren't very happy about the *abruptly* part. They got over it, however, when they realized that I would be giving back every cent I'd made as an employee (plus more) as a frequent and loyal customer throughout my high school and college years. Although their marinade recipe remains shrouded in secrecy to this day, I continue to enjoy a warm friendship with the Ruggieri brothers.

I spent the winter of 1982 as the typical junk-food eating, beer-consuming 17-year-old that can still be found right there at your local high school today. As a student, I treaded water a lot, pulling B's and C's in between bouts of ADD, never quite understanding how subjects like algebra, biology and Spanish were going to come into play in the real world. By this time I'd become friends with a solid group of guys who like me, appreciated parties, girls, sports, music and, you guessed it, eating. My food addiction in my high school days was not lost on my buddies, but they always found a way to joke about it and keep it light. "If you put a hot cheerleader or hot cheeseburger in front of Gary, he'd probably go for the cheeseburger," they joked. While that choice may have been a toss up more times than I care to admit, I'd like to think I would have gone for the girl, at least in theory. We never actually put that one to the test.

My friends Larry, Andy and Eddie joined me for everything, from drunken ice hockey to drunken rock concerts. Early on I firmly rejected the notion of peer pressure and wisely picked my friends, based on the kind of people they were inside. They were great guys who kept their feelings about my declining health to themselves without judgment or discrimination towards my weight. By this time I'd peaked at my highest point ever, somewhere around 205-210 pounds—not exactly svelte for someone 5 feet 9 inches tall. While not exactly morbidly obese, the extra weight gave me the appearance of a chubby kid in serious need of a makeover. My signature "urban camouflage" look consisted of jeans, dark hooded sweaters, concert t-shirts and some kind of baseball hat to top it off. All things considered, I was about as fashionable as the Michelin Tire Man. *Ladies, don't let this one get away!*

As my junior year of high school dragged on, I decided to sign up to play lacrosse, hoping that workouts like the ones the Bull Dog had subjected me to years earlier would send my weight in the right direction. By then, Rainbow and I were having weekly talks about my weight problem. At 17 years of age, I wanted none of it. It was apparent that my mother was on a mission to see me experience life as a thin and healthy guy, but I was far too young and crazy to go join some Weight Watchers chapter again. Occasionally, when my mom could get my friends alone, she would plead with them to keep me from drinking and eating junk food, but alas, my buddies knew I could never truly be policed. "Gee, Mrs. Marino, we'll see what we can do," is how I imagine my friends handled it. That's one part Eddie Haskell, one part Richie Cunningham for those of you following along. Let's face it, folks, when you're a teenager, staging interventions for your friends is hardly on your "things I'd like to do before graduation" list. Picture the scene: *Come on Gary, step away from the pizza, just hand it over to me. You don't want it. This for your own good. We love you man, now hand us the pizza and go with the nice nutritionist here. It's all going to be all right, you'll see.* My friends were not responsible for my health crisis. That's not to say that they didn't care; they were just enjoying being young.

By March of 1982, lacrosse was underway and I was optimistic about becoming the fit and healthy high schooler I'd always wanted to be. Between sprints, laps, running exercises and scrimmages, I began to feel at least some of the weight coming off. By the time the first game kicked off in April, my friends and I had developed a new twist to high school athletics: We drank beers before games and ate at McDonalds before practices. As if my playing on the field wasn't bad enough already, now I was getting buzzed before the games. The junk food intake continued as well, and as the season went on it was apparent that I wouldn't be losing any weight as an active member of the team.

Not long after lacrosse season ended, a new phase in my life began. After only one failed attempt, I successfully got my drivers license. From that day on, the Drive-thru King of the 80's was born. The ability to drive meant I could obtain fast food or any type of food very fast. Food had clearly become my drug, and now I could obtain it any time I wanted to. The independence of having my license was as empowering as it was for any 17-year-old, but for me it essentially turned my car into a buffet on wheels. In fairly short order I became razor sharp at the art of eating and driving. Now, we all do it, but as always, I took it to a "Supersized" level, if you will.

For instance, did you know that traveling at 65 mph, a full sized cinnamon apple crisp can be consumed utilizing your left knee to steer the car and alternating your right hand between the steering wheel and the plastic spoon in the dessert? Kids, don't try this at home, but condiments can be spread on a foot-long hot dog at 45 miles per hour by balancing it on your stomach between your chest and lower belly. Quickly alternate left and right hands while using your teeth to rip the small ketchup and relish packages open. Proceed with caution.

Want more? A pint of Ben & Jerry's ice cream can be consumed in any automobile by keeping one hand on the wheel and eating the top third like a conventional ice cream cone. Now the middle can be eaten by utilizing the squeeze-pop method and forcing the ice cream to the top of the container. For the bottom portion, simply puncture the base and suck on it, much like a traditional ice cream cone. Total time from start to completion? Eighteen miles.

There's also a way to crack lobsters tails using an adjustable steering wheel, but I think you catch my drift.

When summer break came in June, I took a part-time job at a local supermarket, Tony's Food King, and divided my time between playing drums with my band, bowling, and playing drunken basketball with friends. Those activities might lead you to believe that I was just a normal teenager, but a teenager pinching 210 pounds is hardly normal, and the ever-vigilant Rainbow began formulating a plan. Senior year and college awaited, and Rainbow desperately wanted me to experience the life I'd been missing. A new player in the diet industry had quietly come into the area. It was a company called Weight Loss Clinic. Music to Ma's ears, I'm sure. We drove over to their Cambridge offices on a hot day in July of 1982. The walk-in clinic approach was a new one at the time, and in the waiting room before-and-after advertisements were plastered everywhere. Written accounts of individual weight loss war stories were neatly stacked on the tables in front of me. However, there is nothing more inspirational to a 17-year-old than beautiful dieticians, and Weight Loss Clinic had plenty of them. Good concept. It worked for me. I filled out the lengthy paperwork in the lobby while Ma enthusiastically cut a check for the program. My dietitian's name was Nancy or Lisa or something. I was automatically drawn to her gorgeous blue eyes and blond hair. Weight Watchers was never quite like this place. She crafted a low-calorie, low-fat diet for me, consisting of lots of fruits and vegetables and sandwiches with turkey and tuna on extra thin bread. Beer & junk food was to be avoided at all costs. Once my friends realized I was turning over a new leaf, they were immediately supportive. Daily visits to The Weight Loss Clinic, coupled with walks around the lake, was a successful approach, and in no time I was losing four to six pounds a week. Perhaps after spending most of my high school career with a chunky monkey on my back, I was ready to truly get healthy again.

The momentum really picked up in late August as my walks turned to fast jogs. A distinct aura of personal victory began to surface during that summer and I began to feel healthy for the first time since that summer in 1978 when I had joined Weight Watchers. Eventually, I decided it was time for some new clothes to go with my new body, so I headed to the Meadow Glen Mall. There I purchased nylon running suits, dress shirts, painter's pants and a Members Only jacket. Ah, the Eighties…

By September of 1982, after a successful weight loss of thirty-five pounds, a tanned, slimmed-down 175-pound version of Gary Marino appeared in the hallways of good old Medford High. Like a new car, this model was faster, full of flashy upgrades, and handled even better than the last version. The weight loss had an immediate impact on the folks I'd been going to school with for years. "Wow, look at you! How much are you down?" was one enthusiastic reaction. "I was wondering when you'd finally get your act together," was another. "You look great," said one ex-girlfriend. "Could we talk alone sometime?"

The positive reaction to my weight loss was so overwhelming and enthusiastic that it caught even me off guard. I had no idea the impact getting in shape would have on my classmates. The situation was a real eye-opener for me. Apparently my classmates were more attuned to my weight situation and cosmetic looks than I was. I began to get the distinct feeling that they'd written me off as some kind of lost cause, and here I was—svelte, healthy and dressed like "Rick Springfield meets Don Johnson." Bad 80s wardrobe aside, I returned to Medford High victoriously, ready to restart my high school years the way they were meant to be. As I collected high fives and pretty girls' phone numbers in the hallways at school, my mind centered around only one thought: *this is going to be the greatest year of my life!* Unfortunately, that optimism was short-lived, and history was strangely about to repeat itself.

As school got back into swing, my cohorts and I returned to our traditions of drinking, eating and partying. At first, everything was cool. I had the two things I'd always wanted: I had the ability to eat my favorite foods while remaining an aesthetically healthy guy, but the powerful addiction I'd always felt inside was alive and raging. I remember being amazed at how powerful my connection to food still was. As time went on, the beer, pizza, roast beef sandwiches and chocolate chip cookies took their toll. The weight came back on, slowly and subtly. Two pounds this week, three pounds the next week. Then the exercise routine went from five days to two days to non-existent. As with most addicts, I was in denial, thinking I'd put on just a couple of pounds here and there. As my clothes got tighter and that bloated, lethargic feeling returned, I knew in my heart of hearts that the battle was far from over.

By the end of October, the bulk of my thirty-five pound weight loss was back and it was not exactly going unnoticed by my classmates. "Hey, what the hell happened to you? You were looking so good," was one draining comment. "You probably did a lot better with the ladies a couple of months ago," was another. As my senior year unfolded into just another routine year, I did what most food addicts do: I tuned out my physical situation. I paid no attention to my new clothes that now looked ridiculously tight. I ignored my inability to move around physically, turned a blind eye to feeling older than an 18-year-old should feel. I never looked in the mirror below my neck. The emotional blow of gaining the weight back in such a short amount of time put me in a freefall, making me head for the food faster than ever before. My health game was falling like a row of dominos—we're talking pizza here, my friends. Medium, double cheese with onions. Try three times per week, sitting right there in the passenger seat next to me, riding shotgun, like the invisible one I was taking to my head.

I continued, of course, to visit the Weight Loss Clinic almost daily throughout the weight gain, but by this time my enthusiasm lagged and the place seemed to lose its magical *life-makeover* appeal. I'd gone from being the company's poster child to just another weight-loss casualty who had lost the fire. As I write this, a sudden bittersweet feeling comes over me. It occurs to me that it has been over twenty years since I enthusiastically returned to Medford High School to begin that special senior year. Closing my eyes, I recall the feeling of youthful optimism I had as I walked down those hallways, receiving high fives from friends and compliments from supporters. It's September, 1982. I'm the person I've always wanted to be—fit, healthy, energetic and ready to take on the world. For a fleeting moment in time, the road of opportunity and happiness is wide open, with no health obstacle in the way. The scene fades. I'll never know what my life would have been like if that scene had kept right on going. Now it's long past too late, and I can only imagine the possibilities of what my life would have been like over these past two decades.

But back in early 1983, I was still considering drastic measures to put my weight issues behind me. The local Army recruiter had come to our high school to administer the ASCAB tests and after receiving my scores, it seemed that the US Army wanted me—fat or not. Hey, it's always nice to be wanted, right? So I seriously considered a career in the military for three reasons. First, because the recruiter seemed to think I'd make a darned good quota...I mean soldier. Second, because jumping out of helicopters and into the woods with camouflage and advanced weaponry seemed pretty damn cool to me at the time. Third, because I thought the discipline of boot camp, as hard as it would be, might be what I needed to get my health together once and for all. So in May, on the brink of graduation, I visited the local army recruiter in Medford Square. "230 pounds," said the officer as I stepped off the scale. It seemed that I wouldn't be going to boot camp after all. He explained that if I signed the contract (which was right on the table with a new camouflage pen on top), the Army would probably send me to Texas to a special weight-loss camp for two to three months instead. I ask you in all honesty, isn't boot camp hard enough? Now I'm going to "fat" camp boot camp? Suddenly, I had a vision of the Bulldog dressed in green Army fatigues. An obstacle course in Texas on a 98-degree day in July. Me looking like John Candy in the movie "Stripes." "All right, Recruit Marino, line up! You're gonna run! You're gonna swing! Now drop to the ground and give me 20 push-ups. I said go go go go go!" I took a minute to reflect on the situation. Once again, my size was an obstacle to taking the normal steps in life that most people seemed to take. Would it ever end? I took the pen and contract and left the Army Recruiters office with a promise to consider signing within 10 days.

When I returned home, my brother Rich greeted me in the driveway of our home. "Congratulations, brother," he said. You've been accepted at Salem State College." No small feat for a kid with average grades. When I walked through the door a while later, my Mom, always the ultimate cheerleader, enthusiastically greeted me with her trademark warmth and sweet smile. "You'll be the first Marino male to graduate college," she gushed. "Your father will be thrilled!". Ma and I embraced and while we did, I tossed the Army contract into the trash can behind her (I kept the pen). Go to fat camp/boot camp with the Bulldog or make your parents proud? The decision was made right there in my mom's kitchen at that very moment.

Following high school commencement in June, my friends and I made the usual rounds at graduation parties—drinking beers, destroying buffets and chasing girls whom we'd most likely never see again. All of this with Michael Jackson's *Thriller* album blaring in the background. I was enjoying the excesses by this point, with no real plan in place to tackle the 60 pounds of fat that had found its way onto my body over a six-month period. With three months to go before college, I signed up for additional hours at the supermarket, where I'd just been promoted to grocery clerk. Life was sweet, all right, especially when a new rule concerning damaged items was put into place—one that could do no good for anyone struggling with their weight. If a food item was damaged, employees could eat the contents as long as the package was properly placed out back into its respective vendor-credit envelope. Anyone see the problem developing here? We're talking about hungry 18-year-old boys, most of whom have been drinking beer in the parking lot prior to their shift. The back room of the supermarket was full of nooks and closets which soon overflowed with damaged items. Devil Dogs, M&M candies, Flakey Puffs (anyone remember them?), Oreos and bags of assorted mini-chocolate bars. You name it, it was in there. As the storeroom out back began to resemble a temple of sweets, my friends and I were overdosing on sugars. If a manager asked "Can someone get the mop?" eight volunteers would suddenly respond enthusiastically. It's not called stealing, right folks? It's called "sampling the product line." So there we'd all be, in a broom closet somewhere, jamming cupcakes, brownies and assorted nuts into our faces. Leading the charge would be none other than myself, who later took the party to an even more ridiculous level.

Sunday morning was the supermarket cleaning day and employees from all departments were required to be there at 7:00 a.m. to disassemble their individual departments and thoroughly clean them out. Deli, grocery, produce, and so on. Everyone was working hard, but the chief complaint among the employees seemed to be breakfast. During the week we overdosed ourselves on junk food, but Sundays seemed to be a different story. Overworked and still hung over from Saturday night, everyone seemed to be in the mood for a good old-fashioned breakfast.

"Gary, you're a good cook, why can't you figure out how to make us breakfast on Sunday mornings?" they'd ask. Well, that was all the challenge I needed. It was time to get innovative. First, I noticed that the wrapping machines in the meat room had been set to only half of their potential heat temperature. I surmised that if turned up the entire way, they could generate enough heat to actually fry eggs and bacon, which we had readily available in aisle seven. But what about a frying pan? Aisle one took care of that problem. There I found a Jiffy Pop display. I determined that if I scooped out the popcorn kernels but kept the oil base, the round foil container would work nicely. "Ring me up for one of these," I told the girl at the cash register. In aisle six we sold plastic cooking utensils and paper plates. I also found a nice spatula to make omelets. In aisle three were the assorted spices, such as pepper, paprika and so forth. Soon enough our Sunday morning cleaning rituals included country-style breakfasts with omelets made to order. "Who had the ham, cheese and pepper?", I'd yell from my omelet station in the meat room. My co-workers loved it.

"Lisa would like another egg sandwich on raisin toast with butter when you can get to it," they'd call. In the Jiffy Pop containers I'd cook up home-fried potatoes from the produce department and bagels from the deli. Somehow I managed to turn my supermarket gig into a runaway food train again. By the time classes had begun at Salem State College, I was weighing in at a solid 265 pounds. At nineteen years of age, I was starting to feel old before my time.

Right around that time, Rainbow miraculously came up with yet another weight loss program, this one at the Woburn Rehab near Winchester, Massachusetts. As usual, she was more than willing to pay for the costs of the program. Unlike the others I'd been on in the past, the program was headed by a great doctor named Richard Wise, who, following my thorough examination, explained the approach. "We'll have you on two protein shakes per day in place of breakfast and supper," Dr. Wise informed me. "One healthy balanced meal at lunch (today you might call this the Slimfast Diet Plan)." The doctor explained that in addition, there would be sodium tablets and vitamin supplements to take.

Now the word "balanced" meant "boring" to a beer-drinking, junk-food-eating college freshman like me. But while the doctor's diet regimen was hardly music to my ears, I was definitely willing to try anything to avoid spending my college years battling with my weight as I had all through high school. On the positive side, the program did have a refreshing three-point approach, the likes of which I had not seen before. Each week, the 15 or so participants of the weight-loss plan would meet at the Rehab as a group. We'd meet in the waiting room and be individually weighed by a doctor and nurse. Then we'd go over any problems or health concerns we were experiencing. Blood would be checked and weight charts would be updated. Shortly thereafter, the group would file into an adjoining conference room with Dr. Wise and his impressive staff. There we would discuss any psychological issues we were dealing with while trying to stay on the strict program. His team was compassionate and listened well, always giving us appropriate advice on how to handle the tough times. One guy next to me complained that Burger King had come out with a new line of commercials which asked, "Aren't you hungry?" as a massive burger came at the screen. Another talked about how much he missed his wife's award-winning lasagna. *These folks need some serious help,* I thought as I eyed them from across the table. After about 45 minutes, we filed into yet another room. This one was a large workout space with loud music playing. There, a perky aerobics instructor coached us in everything from calisthenics to cardio workouts to light aerobics (which I immediately realized was a lot harder than it looked on television). The program's approach covered the medical, psychological and physical aspects of losing weight. Initially, I had some success on the diet, but the big challenge for me lay in all those college parties I was attending on weekends. I could sacrifice the eating, but how does one not drink? Anyone who has ever attended those campus parties knows exactly what I'm talking about here. It's oceans of beer, a sea of faces, and drinking till you drop. Frankly, you don't *want* to be sober when you see how ridiculously stupid and intoxicated everybody gets. When I brought this dilemma up to the fine staff at the Rehab during our next meeting, they had a creative solution. "Empty out your beer in the bathroom, fill it with water and put your vitamin and sodium tablets (which fizzed like Alka-Seltzer) in the water so it looks like beer," one nurse suggested. *Here we go again.* I laughed. Sound like fun yet? Now I'm to attend parties stone cold sober, passing on my first drug which is food, and faking that I'm actually enjoying my second drug, alcohol. What's next? Should I take an inflatable doll to the parties as my date? *Let the good times roll!*

Well, after about three weeks, my resolve—as you can imagine—began to wane. I'd gone from four or five donuts every morning to a chocolate shake instead. From cheeseburgers every lunchtime to a plain and simple tuna salad. At night a second chocolate shake and some fake beer. One night in January I'd gotten to the Rehab for the meeting a bit early. Half a dozen participants of the program were sitting around in the waiting room, complaining about how hard they were finding the diet. "Well, it wouldn't be so hard if not for my wife's cooking," said one man in his fifties. "She makes a crown pork roast you can only dream about!"

"I love a good pork roast," responded a woman to my right.

"How does she prepare it?" asked another.

"Well, she sautés the potatoes and stuffing in oil and butter and blah blah blah…" responded the man with the talented wife.

The whole time, I'm leaning against a wall, rolling my eyes. "I've got a great recipe for stuffed leg of lamb if you'd like it," said one portly gentleman in a business suit.

My God, I thought, *these people are exchanging recipes in the waiting room of a diet program. Only in America! Maybe I should have gone to Fat Camp/Boot Camp after all,* I thought. I decided to exit the conversation. When I walked around the corner, two older female participants were exchanging numbers and making plans to have dinner at Red Lobster the following week. It didn't seem like anybody was going to have much success on the program at that rate. So following the aerobics workout (I had my eye on the adorable cutie teaching the class), I officially packed it in at the Woburn Rehab. Another diet had ended in failure. Since I'd been denying myself the past month, li'l Gary was looking to settle the score. That's exactly how I looked at it. Everybody I knew had been chowing down around me, and now I was going to get even. I decided to hit every drive-thru, donut shop, buffet and college party I could find. Come to think of it, that actually would have been a nifty time for my friends to start in on that food intervention.

As my teenage years wound down, like most overweight people, I began to invite denial into my brain. *Even if I'm not successful at getting this weight off, I know modern science is developing a drug right now.* In my mind I truly believed that somewhere in some government laboratory, scientists were gorging themselves on pizza and Chinese food and then popping pills into their mouths just to experiment with their new anti-fat drug. As a frustrated nineteen-year-old, I was ready and willing to be the first in line for the "magic bullet" clinical trials. Did they need a guinea pig? No problem. I eagerly surfed TV channels, expecting to stumble upon the press conferences I knew had to be going on somewhere. "We're making great progress on a fat burning drug. Until then, keep your chins up!"

I held faith that I'd see the day, and see it soon, when that magic pill would be released over the counter. Maybe it would burn the fat while I slept. Perhaps it could neutralize the calories before they could be processed in the body. No matter what, I was sure at some point "it" was coming. As far as I was concerned, if in 1983 we could make Michael Jackson look like a werewolf, surely in 1984 we could make a guy like me look physically fit.

1984. What a year! The country was enjoying a boom economy, Ronald Reagan had everyone feeling patriotic, and the Boston Celtics had once again become World Champions. In our world, the Marino family was gearing up for my sister Donna's marriage to her high school sweetheart and champion hockey player, Tony Miller. On TV, a handsome young man named Mark Hughes was passionately and enthusiastically peddling his diet product known as Herbalife. In shrewdly produced infomercials—a relatively new concept at the time—Hughes stood on stage in front of packed audiences telling his story. At first glance, I had to admit it was rather compelling. Hughes's mother had suffered a life-long weight problem. Growing up, he had helplessly watched as she became the guinea pig for one scam diet product after another. Eventually, the overdose of diet pills and fad diets permanently damaged her health and in 1972, young Mark Hughes became a boy without a mother. He'd made it his life's mission to avenge her death by inventing a safe, effective weight loss solution for the masses. Hughes studied the healing power of natural herbs. He partnered with schools and herbal specialists and patented his product. A weight loss dynasty was born. The one-hour plus infomercials had all the glory of a Republican National Convention (which was occurring just a few channels down) and Hughes appeared to be funny, charming and genuine.

As we watched the TV, Ma addressed me with a serious concern of hers. "Your sister's wedding is coming up and the tuxedos Tony picked out don't run in big sizes," she pleaded. "Please, if not for yourself, then for me, try to lose some weight before the wedding."

Now as an usher, I had to admit it would look pretty bad to wear a different style tux from the rest of the wedding party. Rainbow had a point. By now the pleading routine had gotten old, but that mother of mine was one sweet woman. As far as I was concerned, she deserved nothing but svelte, polished, healthy and successful kids. The team player that she was, Ma offered to go on the product with me, so I decided to give the fine folks at Herbalife a shot. Talk about deja diet: two shakes a day, one sensible meal, and in between, an energy tablet called NRG. Pretty original, huh? NRG, according to the infomercial, was made from ancient Indian herbs and caused an abundance of energy. I remembered NRG the first time it came out, back when it was known as 'speed.' Well, from the looks of me a few days later, whizzing up the four flights of stairs to class at Salem State, you could be sure that the NRG product worked. But significant weight loss still seemed to elude me on the Herbalife diet plan. Maybe it was the chalky-tasting shakes. All the blended bananas in the world couldn't change that consistency. Or perhaps the problem was that my one meal each day consisted of a large roast beef and cheese grinder with mustard and mayo (I'd been transferred to the deli department at Tony's Food King by that time). It also may have been that the dozens of Herbalife distributors calling me to join their distribution sales pyramids were turning me off to the diet completely. Whatever it was, I knew my days on Herbalife were numbered. At that point in my life, I was just a kid who wanted to enjoy being a college sophomore. The diet game was getting old, and my Herbalife Shakes were beginning to look like just another chapter in a long, drawn-out saga of a lifelong food addict. Now all of these fad diets and their ill effects on my body would come with a price in the years to come, but at the time I was young, energetic and had time on my side.

Predictably, when the October wedding rolled around, I was struggling to fit into the slick tuxedo my future brother-in-law had picked out. For a time I considered going for the Miami Vice style tuxes, which did run in my size, but then it occurred to me how blatant that would have been. The "big guy" in a screaming pastel tux, while the rest of the wedding party wore black. As usual, my folks dipped into their pockets again to have a talented tailor named Marco let the tux out in all the right places. With a bruised ego and an altered tuxedo, I ushered family and friends down the church aisle on a picture-perfect day in October, 1984. The happy couple exchanged nuptials and threw one of the best weddings ever. A six-piece band called "Rocky Road" got the crowd jamming and on the dance floor. Despite being aerodynamically challenged, I ripped one up for the men of girth out there, utilizing moves even *I* didn't know I had. My folks lovingly watched their kids and basked in the glow of the day's events. Today my sister and her husband are still happily married and have four beautiful and intelligent kids. Watching their family is like watching ours all over again. Even better, as they are all fit, healthy and enjoying their lives everyday. Sometimes life can be a beautiful thing.

Back in 1985, however, my life was still about the quest for health. I heard about a hypnosis specialist in Arlington by the name of Andson Verner. He'd apparently been successful in helping folks quit smoking as well as overeating, and a friend suggested I schedule a session with him at his Universal Hypnosis Center. Sounds impressive, doesn't it?

I walked up three flights of stairs on a Monday night in 1985 and met Andson at the top step. He was around 60 years of age with thick, uncombed gray hair and a loud, almost hypnotizing plaid suit.

"Pleased to meet you. Come in, come in!" Andy said as he handed me his business card. Right away I knew I was in trouble. The card was a loud yellow and orange kaleidoscope design with white lettering. It was so dizzying to look at, I couldn't take my eyes off of it. Unfortunately, that would be the closest I would come to being hypnotized that night. Mr. Verner had me sit in a comfortable

Lazy Boy chair with my feet up. New Age music played softly in the background. *Okay, let's have it,* I sarcastically thought. *Where is it? I know it's coming. Where's the cheesy fake gold pocket watch that goes back and forth in front of my face?* "I want you to keep your eyes on this pocket watch," he said a second later. *Ah, there it was.* From there we went through the whole clichéd hypnosis routine. "Gary, I want you to count down from 50," he intoned. "I want you to go to a warm, safe place in your mind where you feel relaxed. Are you there Gary?"

"Yep," I answered.

"Where is that place?" he asked.

"Well, right about now I'm in a Burger King drive-thru, Mr. Verner." End of session. As I drove home from my hypnosis session to stop overeating, I purchased a Big Mac and fries from McDonald's for the ride home, wondering what the next pathetic chapter of my weight-loss saga would be.

Right around that time, my dad, frustrated from years of watching me struggle with my food addiction (and perhaps even more frustrated watching my mom get depressed about it), came to me with the answer to all my problems.

"I saw this infomercial late last night with people listening to these subliminal audio tapes and losing weight," he said. "People were swearing by them. They were expensive, but I ordered them because it's time to take care of this once and for all." *Here we go again,* I remember thinking. *People thinking it's just as easy as a swipe of the credit card to fix the problem. But hey, people on the paid advertisement were swearing by it, right?* I thanked my father and waited for the tapes to arrive. Three days later a UPS shipment came to the door. In it were dozens of tapes, labeled with names like "Stopping Bingeing" and "The Power Of Positive Eating." I slipped the Van Halen cassette out of my Walkman and inserted the tape labeled something like "Curbing Your Subconscious Appetite." Mystical music came on, with an announcer with an FM radio-type voice telling me that I didn't need to overeat anymore. I was the most important person in the world. I was capable of taking lemons and making lemonade. I was not a loser; I was a loser in transition. The tapes went on and on about putting myself first and realizing what an incredible person I truly was. Well, three days of listening to these tapes had me feeling like a complete egomaniac. I wasn't losing any weight or curbing my eating. However, I had no doubt that I, in fact, was "the most important person in the world." I shoved the tapes back into the box and jammed them into the back of my closet. Dad seemed surprised and disappointed that the tapes hadn't done the trick. I desperately wanted my father to realize that he couldn't buy my health for me. I wanted him to see that what I was going through was like nothing he had ever experienced. In the end, I realized that in his lifetime he would probably never understand what an overweight person like me was going through.

That's when my first experience with the concept of therapy began. By the fall of 1986, depression seeped into my life for the first time. I wasn't quite sure what was happening to me, but years of losing at the weight game had me feeling stuck in life and this attitude began to affect me in a negative way. A dark sensation seemed to orbit my mind, washing over me like storm clouds. Textbook depression had set in, along with the helpless feeling of being trapped. Years later I would be told it was low-level depression brought on by my food addiction—a situation many lifelong addicts experience. We're not talking genetically-induced family depression, but depression brought on by addiction, the feeling of being trapped in your own body and losing at the losing game. *Kids, don't let this happen to you* type stuff. My folks noticed the personality change and scheduled a sit-down session with a psychologist named Dr. Sigel. I wasn't sure what to expect from therapy in terms of actual help, but one thing was sure: the stigma of needing a shrink was only adding to my already low self-esteem.

I met with the good doctor weekly from the fall of 1986 through the summer of 1987. I immediately took a liking to him, but as we talked about my life and problems, it occurred to me that in my darkest hour he couldn't help me understand why I overate or became depressed. Poor guy. Maybe he was in over his head. Or perhaps I was simply too embarrassed and therefore hiding my true feelings, giving him little to work with. Whatever it was, Dr. Sigel was the type of guy I would have liked to hang out and have a beer with—low-key, interesting and very cool—but I figured I had friends with whom I could talk about my problems, and at $90 a session, I decided to move on. When the therapeutic approach didn't yield any results, it occurred to me that in all likelihood my college years would mirror my high school years. I began to question the meaning of it all. Was this what I was meant to be like? At times, I'd put on a good face, ignore my weight, and try to live life to its fullest. If only back then I'd been able to foresee what was to come, perhaps I'd have tried just a little bit harder to honestly work on dissecting my food addiction.

Rainbow was the next one to step up to the plate with a short-lived solution to my weight problem. She called me for a sit-down one Saturday morning in the early spring and pleaded with me to join the local chapter of Overeaters Anonymous. *Anonymous* I thought? *Isn't it a little late for that? Everyone knows I'm a walking Super Bowl Party.* Rainbow explained that she felt it might be time to turn to God to help put an end to my food issues, and this was the basis for the Overeater Anonymous' 12-step program. I rejected the concept immediately on the basis that I hadn't been to church since I had graduated from St. Joseph's Grammar School.

"I think you need help from a higher power," said my mother. Just as I was about to roll my eyes and tell her that I was enjoying being a twenty-two-year old beer-drinking, late-night chicken-finger-eating college hell raiser, I looked deep into my mother's eyes. There was concern and pain in them. I had put undo stress on her for the better part of a decade. Years of living this disease with her son and seeing him endure the effects of food addiction had taken a toll on my mom. Although I didn't want to admit it, a big part of me was also desperate for help. But a religious approach? "Religion and a sponsor," she informed me. They assign you a sponsor for support. Someone you can call whenever you feel the need to overeat. "He'll check in with you every day as well," she said.

"You mean, like this dude will call me here?" I asked with declining interest. "And will he bring me take-out food when I fall off the wagon?" I took an even longer second look at my mother's face in an attempt to make sense of these familiar conversations—conversations that had become a significant part of our relationship. Rainbow looked older to me now, and as I searched deeper into her eyes, I could see the years of worrying I had caused her because of my declining health. These should have been normal conversations between a mother and her son: issues about grades and girls, not God and girth. I knew one thing for sure: that woman deserved better.

So on a Sunday morning in April of 1987, I reluctantly woke up early and headed for my first Overeaters Anonymous meeting at a hospital in Medford. Right off the bat, the "early on Sunday" thing had me in a bad frame of mind as I entered the parking lot and headed, with other super-heavies, up a hill and into the meeting room. Needless to say, college age kids are all about sleeping off hangovers on Sundays, right?

When I entered the main building where the meeting was to take place, I slowly made my way up the center isle in a room overflowing with church-like pews. It was quite an appropriate theme, in retrospect. Almost immediately I found myself put off by the scene around me. Everybody in the place was huge. I mean *Honey I blew up the people in the steeple* huge. *I don't belong here,* I remember thinking. *A guy could develop a mental hang up.* As I searched for a seat, I noticed something peculiar and yet almost comical. Everyone, and I mean *everyone* in the place was breathing heavy. Now 150 wheezing heavy breathers made me want to head for the door, but the look in my mother's eyes once again came to mind and I sat down like a man whose spirit had been broken. A short, thin, bald man with a beard and plaid shirt stepped up to a podium and kicked off the meeting.

"Hello, everyone, I'm Jerry," he said. "I'm 41 years old, and before I came here I had a $30-a-day Chinese food habit." An audible "ooohhh" and "ahhhh" rushed through the crowd and I turned around in my seat, taking in the scene around me. People were glued to Jerry's story. *Sign on as my sponsor, Jerry,* I thought. *I'll have you up to $60 per day.* Jerry went on to chronicle his battles with Kung Pao Chicken and his run-ins with Pork Low Mein. With each story of Egg Foo Yung and Beef Chow Yoke, the crowd responded with an enthusiastic, "We love you, Jerry!" Everyone except me. I responded by stopping, dropping, and rolling towards the door. Grown men crying over spilled moo shi pork really left me cold. I would not spend quality sleeping time on Sundays with a room full of heavy breathers who, in my opinion, were clearly in much more trouble than I was in terms of their addictions. "These people are in extreme trouble," I said to myself as I slammed the doors open on the way to the parking lot. If only that morning I'd made the connection between the Overeaters Anonymous crowd and the empty take-out bag of Chinese food containers in my back seat, perhaps I'd have gone back in. Instead, I headed back to bed, some might say for the better part of a decade. In all fairness, Overeaters Anonymous has helped thousands of people for many years, and maybe if I had realized that I would be struggling with this addiction for the next fifteen years, I would have made Kung Pao Jerry my personal sponsor.

By 1987, part time jobs in the food industry had begun to bore me. The diet counselor I'd been seeing at the Weight Loss Clinic in Cambridge suggested that I work in a setting outside of the food industry. That was sound advice. Where that advice was 5 years earlier, I had no idea. I decided to try something in line with my media/communications major at Salem State College.

KISS 108 FM was America's original super-radio station. It started in 1979 as a disco station right in my own hometown of Medford, and by the early 1980s was one of the most influential Top 40 stations in the country. The success was due in part to Sunny Joe White, a program director and larger-than-life on-air personality who had developed a creative adult contemporary format. The successful on air music mix included oodles of national and local celebrities, often with sports stars guest hosting and making appearances. KISS was a very cool place to work at the time. Every three-piece-suited record executive followed by every one-hit wonder seemed to walk through those doors. There were the Milli Vanilli guys on Monday, followed by Huey Lewis on Tuesday, Valerie "Van Halen" Bertinelli on Wednesday, the Miami Vice guys on Thursday and a legend like Smokey Robinson on Friday. Even a big guy like me could get an esteem boost coming into contact with stellar company like that. The innovative format truly was "Entertainment Radio." Sunny, along with the station owner Richard Balsbaugh, shrewdly engineered the annual KISS Concerts, where as many as 40 national recording stars would descend on Boston to play live and raise money for children's charities. The shows were knockouts and garnered national media attention. No radio station at the time had produced live shows of such caliber. As a result, each and every spring, for one weekend only, Boston was transformed into Hollywood East. You name the celebrity, and they were right there at KISS every year: Cher, Whitney Houston, Elton John, Rod Stewart, David Lee Roth, Will Smith, Meat Loaf, Heart, Brian Adams, Aerosmith and on and on and on.

A friend of the family managed to get me an internship, which was not easy to do at that time. KISS was impressive and everyone wanted in. I got along well with Sunny and most of the other jocks almost immediately. The station seemed to attract two types of employees: good looking people who were successful or good looking people who looked successful. Everybody was buff, well-dressed and into style and fashion. Well, in America you never get a second chance to make a first impression, and mine was apparently blown the day I walked through the door. Most of the sales people, as well as the programmers, treated me well. But in a fairly short amount of time I was enduring the lengthy dieting talks that had followed me my entire life, like "You should eat lots of pasta, and keep fresh fruit in a bag in your locker." Of course ten years later, Dr. Robert Atkins would be shooting holes in that advice. Then there was the second-hand advice: "Have you considered joining a liquid diet program? So & so at the oldies station across town just lost a ton of weight on one." That's some good advice, right? "Just don't eat for a few months and you'll be fine." Finally there was the fanatical advice. "I've got a brother who was once twice as big as you and he lost it on a grapefruit diet. You like grapefruit?" I remember thinking, *God, are these new life-architect types beginning to bore me.* I'd just "yes" them to death and go on with my business.

Meanwhile, invitations to record label parties, pre-concert bashes or staff parties where food, booze and drugs were all over the place flowed into the station. By the end of 1987 I'd begun working on the nighttime radio programs. It was there that I noticed an interesting trend. Restaurants from all over the greater Boston area were sending complimentary food to the nighttime jocks with the hope of scoring free radio plugs, and in true food addict form, I began to manipulate it for my own benefit. The cost of a 30-second spot at that time was out of reach for most local restaurants, but the restaurant owners knew that their costs for half a dozen complimentary dinners were next to nothing. By this time I'd bonded with the nighttime disc jockeys over our mutual love of food, so they were more than happy to let me spin my magic. I simply reversed the process. Instead of waiting for restaurant people to show up, I put a 'food for plugs' type of system into place. I'd pull out the phone book and call them. "Hi, this is Gary over at KISS 108, and I'd like to order..." Right about that point in the conversation they'd usually cut me off. "KISS 108, wow!" they'd interject. "Hey, how does this sound? We'll send some free dinners if you just say 'hi' to us and thank us on the air."

"Sounds like a plan," I'd respond. "Just send us more of whatever you sent us two nights ago." Like some sort of food mafia, you name it, we had it. Mouthwatering Thai food, a dozen hot Chicken Kabob dinners, 20 heaping BLT sandwiches, they all lined up in the on-air studio like a company cookout. A smorgasbord of pizzas with assorted toppings...And so, 10 years after my friends and I took the Bean Villa down for the count, I was still in the free food business. It was like some sort of black market and I milked it for all it was worth. The disc jockeys would marvel at my ability to work my magic with the local restaurants and the poor morning show crew would smell BBQ dinners at 6:15 am. Occasionally, on my way to school, I heard them talk about it on the air. "Hey, does anybody smell that smell?" they questioned. "What the hell went on in here last night?" I'd chuckle to myself. Well Gar...there you go again. Somehow food had followed me into yet another chapter of my life and the pounds piled on steadily. My weight during that time topped off at around 290 pounds. Unfortunately, the nighttime jocks and their studio help began packing on the pounds as well, but it never seemed to stop them from enthusiastically greeting me with, "Hey Buddy, what're we ordering for the show tonight?" You knew I was working one of the nighttime shows when the disc jockey could barely speak into the microphone to plug an upcoming song because he or she was chewing on some sort of chow. Over time, I fine-tuned the system to the point where I didn't even have to place a specific food order. Just call, mention KISS and prepare for delivery. The leftovers all came home or were tossed out. The sight of all those food platters laid out next to each other in the on-air studio captured the excesses of the radio perk frenzy.

By the spring of 1988, as I always seemed to do in my life, I was taking things from over the top to just plain ridiculous. Once I even booked myself, a fellow producer, and a nighttime disc jockey for a personal appearance at an ice cream joint in Malden Mass. In hindsight, booking the job was probably the beginning of my career as an agent, but back in July of 1988 I was in it for all the wrong reasons. The deal I cut was sweet. We would all be paid an appearance fee in exchange for making a "celebrity" appearance of scooping ice cream for station fans. We'd call a live plug into the radio station, something like, "C'mon down to Mann's Dairy Barn; we'll be scooping ice cream and giving away tee shirts all afternoon". To top it off, the store agreed to send ice cream sundaes and shakes to our radio show for the remainder of the summer. Ridiculous, I know, but by this point I was in a free-fall again. There's a photo at the station to this day of the three of us outside the place, holding ice cream scoops and wearing our foolish "Mann's Dairy Barn" smocks. Hanging behind us are KISS Tee shirts, autographed by a legitimate radio personality and two unknown wise guys. Forget Jerry's Kids; in the photo we looked more like Ben & Jerry's Kids. The episode, although innocent enough from a distance, taught me just how far a food addict will go for half a dozen assorted ice cream flavors per night.

While we're on the subject of ice cream flavors, let me address one thing that I think frozen dessert manufactures need to think about. Studies show that most Americans eat ice cream when they are emotional or having a moment of anxiety. Why then aren't flavors named appropriately? *I'll have a pint of the Financial Crunch please, and a half gallon of Emotional Cripple Ripple. How much for the Chocolate Chip On My Shoulder?*

The Art Of:
THE BIG AND TALL STORE

"Put on a suit. Remember, you can never dress up a fat man too much!"

—Uncle Dave

By the late 1980s I was no stranger to the place where the mannequins have double chins, otherwise known as the Big & Tall Store. It was the premiere experience for guys who were losing the battle of the bulge. Walking into one for the first time was proof positive that you had surrendered too many times. "They hang the clothes on meat hooks in these places," I remember joking on the air during my short-lived radio career at KISS-FM. Of course by this time in my life, self-deprecating humor was the name of the game, and I was serving it up large just to avoid having yet another heart-to-heart talk with concerned family and friends about my ballooning weight problem.

A fairly new chain opened in the Boston area called "Big & Tall/Casual Male." They were beginning to carve quite a niche for themselves, creating colorful, hip and stylish clothes for the "big guys" out there. Today they even have their own newspaper available in the stores called the *Think Big Times*. As a retailer, they were doing a nice job, considering that up until their arrival on the scene folks like myself in the Brotherhood of the Big and Tall were all stuck with bland, overpriced cuts of colorless clothing, including pants with elastic waistbands (not the most attractive look) and wide pants cuffs right out of a 1978 New York disco. You see, the cut was really what was important, and the majority of designers could never seem to grasp the concept that just because a guy had a 58-inch waist didn't mean he had legs like a tree trunk. A guy could be big around the middle but normal everywhere else. Whether you had the *apple* body or the *pear* body, BIG & TALL/Casual Male had your body type covered. Moreover, one look around and you knew these designers had a sense of humor. After all, who else could come up with the name "Himalaya" for a Size 3X Hawaiian shirt? Or how about a 4X size sweater with the brand name "Nights Of The Round Table." *I'll take these two and an order of bruised ego to go, please.* One day I came across one particular garment named "Zeppelin," a 5X double-knit plaid type of thing. As I tried it on, I could actually picture in my mind the workers in the sweatshops, high-fiving each other as they came up with the names. "Let's call this one Everest! Yeahhh!" More high-fiving. *Thanks folks, it's so encouraging to be thought of as a mountain.*

More chains cropped up in the 1990s, and by that time I was in no position to be picky about the brand names. One time I tried on a $400 suit with a size 60-inch waist and a 58-inch jacket. The tailor was on his knees with chalk, marking where the alterations on the dark blue suit needed to be done. Four hundred dollars and the salesman blurts out "after another $60 worth of alterations it will be looking good." I looked down at him piercingly and sarcastically thought, *Pal this was never about looking "good". There's nothing "good" you can do for me here. There are three other suits in my closet right now that don't fit, and even if they did they wouldn't look "good" either. I am here because a man in America, overweight or not, must have a minimum of one suit in case someone dies or gets married. That's why I'm here. I could spend $1,000 on a suit in your store and it wouldn't matter. I'm over 300 pounds, and the issue of looking good was over long before I walked through your door. Surely you've got to know that I can stroll out of this store right now, wearing a $5,000 Armani suit and what people on the street will see is a man who they think cares about nothing, including himself. A bloated aberration of a human with absolutely no love for his body or himself. Maybe they'll know me, maybe they won't, but that's what they will see. So let's keep the words "looking good" out of the conversation.* But what came out of my mouth was, "Here's my credit card."

I'm baring my soul a bit here, but this truly was my reality. In my humble opinion, anyone in the U.S.A. with a weight problem is fooling himself if he believes he can wear a suit from the Men of Girth Collection and actually look good. Then again, it wasn't all bad shopping at the Casual Male/Big & Tall. That's where I purchased my most colorful bathing suit to date—an electric blue Speedo with pastel patches of green and hot pink all over it—and just to make it a tad bit louder, a nuclear fish pattern ran right through it. "Over the top" was how my Uncle David described the skintight suit, and I quickly dubbed it my "power-packed tropical." The bathing suit became an omen to my friends and family that a silly day of fun in the sun, boating or swimming was in the works at places like Cape Cod, Massachusetts or Marco Island, Florida. "You bring the barbeque, I'll bring the marinated steak tips and power-packed tropical!" I'd call. You see, among friends and in a private ocean setting, a 300+ pound man wearing a retina-damaging tropical bathing suit was pretty darned funny. In public, of course, I wouldn't be caught dead wearing it.

Besides my "power-packed tropicals," the Big & Tall shop provided the setting for one of the funniest situations I can remember. One spring day my friend Jim and I bumped into each other in the Mall parking lot, both heading in the direction of the store. Apparently Jimmy had also been buying his clothes there, but not for the same reason. At 6 feet 8 inches and 180 pounds, he was clearly in it for the "Tall" stuff. Jim revealed to me that he'd been shopping there for quite some time, but dreaded the store manager's "hard sell" approach. "The two of us walking in together would be this guy's dream sale," Jim speculated. I knew the particular manager whom he was talking about. The guy could truly talk a hungry dog away from a flame-broiled steak. We'd conceded that he would make the whole clothes-shopping process pretty painful. I was clearly very *big*. Jim was obviously very *tall*. The two of us quickly came up with a plan.

When we walked through the door, the hawk-like sales manager quickly rushed to the front of the store like a magnet to steel.

"What can I help you fellas with today?" he gleefully asked. The dollar signs and Christmas bonus were so apparent in his eyes you could just see it. We were a dream duo. The Big & Tall chain's target market was standing right in the doorway, and this guy couldn't control his excitement any longer.

Then Jim dropped the bomb. "We're here to shop for a birthday gift for our boss," Jim said. "He's 5'5" and 165 pounds. What have you got?" Big guys 1. Sales guy 0. Mark that on your score cards.

WAISTED YOUTH

"Don't let my glad expression give you the wrong impression"

—*Smokey Robinson, "The Tears of a clown"*

So why is growing up overweight and addicted to food a wasted youth? Well, let's put it this way. Think of all the things you know you need in order to have a successful childhood and young adulthood. Physical and mental health? Absolutely. Self-esteem? It is essential to developing properly. Self-love? Whitney Houston sang about it in "The Greatest Love Of All." Without it, you spend your daily existence daydreaming about having someone else's life. Now personally, I think Whitney could use a little more of it herself these days, but I digress.

Let's break it down even further. When kids tease you or you experience discrimination from family or friends at an early age you never develop a sense of self-worth. When you can't physically excel at sports, games, or competitions because you are carrying too much weight on your body, you begin to develop an inferiority complex. You start to wonder if you are good at anything. Simple motivational building experiences such as winning a sports trophy never happen. Instead, if you're like me, you rack up a small shelf of "Perseverance Awards." Better known as the "He Tried" award. When you grow up without feeling energetic or healthy, it begins to affect your mental outlook and how positively or negatively you see things as well. The only pleasure you get from life is the one that never lets you down: food. It's the gift that keeps on giving, at least until you're incapacitated. This isn't rocket science here—just the facts. When you can't perform well mentally or physically, you're not living a quality life. As the years go by and a fat child develops into a fat adult, key experiences (experiences one needs to have to fully understand life) never happen.

Love, for instance. If you never experience relationships, even innocent pre-teen dating, you can't become a young adult who knows what it is you are looking for in a partner. Being dumped, rejected or broken-hearted (as hard as those experiences are), are feelings that a young person needs to experience in life. Without experiencing both the joys and pains of love, an individual's growth is seriously compromised.

You know what else can become compromised? Your wardrobe. It's not as important as compromising relationships, but certainly it is an issue. When you grow up overweight, you never fit into what everybody else is wearing. Your entire style comes down to what's least objectionable. "Off the rack" rarely happens and you breathe a sigh of relief at just being able to find a pair of "Husky" pants that actually fit. You never shop at places like Gentlemen's Wearhouse because you think it's some sort of exotic dance club of questionable character. You never look in the mirror. You never learn how to be fashionably dressed. And if you're like me, you end up a man in his 30s who thinks GQ stands for Gourmet Quality. While we're on the subject, am I the only person who thinks Giorgio Armani is one of the Three Tenors?

Now not every person who has grown up overweight and food-addicted will agree with my assessment that it is a "waisted youth." Just as the world will always have its Oprahs, Pavarottis and Rosanne Barrs (people who defied their weight problems), it will always have overweight young people who will tell you their youths were not wasted. If they can truly say that, then I'm happy for them. I, for one, do not believe it is possible. Why? Because even if you are a young, overweight person who excels at school, sports, friendships or whatever, it is still impossible to escape the inevitable health problems as well as the constant negative feedback from people around you. Take a walk on a crowded public beach in July. Even if you can handle the mental daggers and verbal S.C.U.D. missiles you'll endure, I'll guarantee that when you head home, family and friends will still make comments, although in a much gentler and more loving way.

Food addiction and obesity lead to a "waisted youth" because we live in a country where political correctness is lost on people of size. Blacks are now African-Americans. The homeless are now practically referred to as professional window-cleaning technicians. But don't wait around expecting the 60+ percent of Americans who are fat to be referred to as "aerodynamically challenged." We're simply fat, right? I believe that as a people, we not only use people's weight problems as the scapegoat for other issues, but we have formed a culture that is tactless in its approach to the overweight population. Allow me to explain. The comments I'm talking about here aren't limited just to me. You hear it happening all around us at any minute. No issue showcases human ignorance more than obesity. Dr. Lee Kaplan of the Mass General Weight Loss center calls it "the last allowable prejudice." On the streets and in the media, the cheap shots are all around us every day. Just listen to some of the morning show disc jockeys right here in Boston or in your hometown. You know, the ones who fawn all over their guests when they're on the air and then throw cheap shots at their weight problems before they've left the lobby. These spineless radio types have never had the problem, but you can bet they'll be reincarnated as 600-pound individuals in their next lives. If you read anger in my words it's because a lifetime of this takes its toll and people need to see through their ignorance at some point in their lives. Obviously I'm a lot more sensitive to people's feelings after having battled this disease. By the same token, I've got to be honest. If I had been successful in my radio career and never battled a weight problem, you'd still never have heard me treating people like that. There's entertainment and there's human decency. Someday the radio show, like your existence, ends and your ratings are scrutinized by a more important boss. It doesn't take a genius to understand this concept, yet compassion is always somehow lost on people whenever it comes to the "fat" thing.

At virtually every phase of my life, the issue of my size dominated my conversations with people. It was a bizarre way to grow up, to say the least. From that day when I was 10, playing football on Mrs. Harrigan's lawn, through junior high, high school, then college and all the way up to building my business and being a guy in his 30s writing a self-help book, my weight has always been front and center wherever human interaction has lurked. These conversations generally fell into three categories:

1. Supporters, concerned family and friends who just wanted to see me get the monkey off my back and get healthy.

2. Deserters, people who once fell into the supporter category, but just could not understand the complexity of the problem. Eventually they got in my face, became angry and frustrated about it, and then went on with their lives and considered me a lost cause.

And 3. Mr. Wonderfuls. You know these guys—the ones who live in the gym by day and call attention to themselves by insulting the not-so-buff people by night. Memo to those guys: "Get over yourselves." Your bodies might be temples, but without heart they're just empty shacks.

Supporters come from all walks of life. They are individuals like my family members, close buddies, or co-workers. Their intentions are always pure and put forth with my health and quality of life interests in mind. "You've got to lose this weight," my mom would say. "You'll never be [insert any age here] again."

When we were alone, my high school or college buddies would hit me with something like, "Dude, I'm just telling you for your own good, you should really try to lose some of that weight." Of course while they were telling me this I'd be drinking an Herbalife Weight Loss Shake while my Lean Cuisine Frozen Dinner was heating up in the oven.

"Any program you want, we'll pay for it," I remember my folks saying.

"You know it doesn't matter to me what size you are, but you really should try..." was one fleeting girlfriend's plea.

My grandfather actually started as a Supporter and went over to the Deserters. From age 13 through 18 he would hit me with lines like, "I'm just telling you because I care," or "You'd be a good-lookin' kid if you'd just lose that weight." Later he became a Deserter. From age 18 through 28, whenever I walked into a room his opening line would be a sarcastic, "You're looking good, kid," or "Keep eating and I'll have to take you to Omar The Tent Maker to buy by your clothes." Thanks, Grampa; I'll just head right up to therapy now. The ironic part was that as he was saying this, my grandmother would be in the other room preparing a crown roast or lasagna to die for. Such a strange way to grow up.

Deserters were always interesting to me. They'd either get mad and in my face or let me know how I was blowing it by not even trying (I was trying, 24/7) or they'd quietly look at me and shake their heads, then distance themselves from me. For whatever reason, I always had plenty of people around, so it never bothered me as much as it could have.

In a lot of ways, Deserters treated my addiction like that of an alcoholic. *He's a good guy, but he can't get that monkey off his back; I hope he figures it all out.*

Mr. Wonderfuls have to draw attention to their own physiques by taking a shot at someone else's. The only way they can shine a little spotlight on themselves is by becoming verbal snipers. "Don't you love your body, man?" said one, as he flexed his muscles at me back in high school.

"Right now I'd love you to [insert insult here]," I came back with. Of course it's bad enough being verbally assaulted by some Mr. Wonderful in your teens or early twenties. Imagine how nauseating it is when you're 29 years old and heading for 30. By then you simply have no tolerance for insults by idiots because you're a grown adult with real responsibilities like anyone else.

Once, while I was walking the historic Minute Man Trail in Lexington, MA, I decided to take my sweater off. The weather had heated up and I was getting hot. As I peeled off my top, a verbal sniper drove by, almost as if on cue. "Put it back on!" he yelled from his car.

Okay, first let's just address this spineless business of yelling out of a moving vehicle. If you feel the need to comment on something you know nothing about to a person you've never met, find a parking space and lay it on the line. That way you at least admit that you are a bit more than a coward. I'll even spring for the meter. Once you've approached the person and returned home, you might even begin to self analyze for the very first time in your life, a process you've obviously been deluding yourself about. Let's take a closer look at the other situation here. What you've got is a heavy guy, clearly dressed in sweatpants, walking in the woods because he knows he needs to lose weight and get healthy. I'm not walking with a pint of Häagen dazs. Besides, if I was, you'd keep your mouth shut because you know it would end up on your windshield or in your face. I was walking that day because I *had* self analyzed and made a decision to vigorously battle my disease, but for some Mr. Wonderful out there, that's apparently not enough. Let's yell out of a moving car because big is, well, *big*. Excuse me. I was unaware I needed your permission, pal. After the unsolicited drive-by commentary, I continued walking along the trail, with a smile permanently implanted on my face. It occurred to me how lucky I was in life. I was merely born with a food addiction. That guy was clearly born without some essential genes. I'll take my lot in life anytime over that guy's.

Supporters, Deserters and Mr. Wonderfuls. Some days I'd actually get hit with all three at once. In the morning, a Supporter. "You should really try to get that weight off; you'll feel a lot better." In the afternoon at work or school, a Deserter. "It's too bad you can't get control; you're a good guy, but you've got to get a clue one of these days." And in the evening, the S.C.U.D. missile compliments of some Mr. Wonderful. "You think you're big? I got a brother twice as fat as you." Thanks, pal. I really feel much better, thanks to that startling revelation. From time to time I'd encounter a supporter who, quite frankly, shouldn't have been a supporter. My best friend's 250-pound grandmother, for instance, who would walk up to me at every family party, take me by the hands while I was at the buffet table and say in broken English "I'ya remeba howa hard it wasa backa whena I'ya wasa overweighta." *Thanks Grandma. By chance, have you been on a scale since you left the old country?*

While I'm on a rant here, there is one other category I haven't mentioned. We'll call these types the Condescending & Cowardly, the folks who take a dig at you without having the guts to say it directly to you. "Hey, it's the Big Guy," they'd say in that underhanded cowardly tone. It's called "hiding a deliberate dig because you don't have the spine to say it for real." We all know this one. You're at a party and in front of an entire crowd someone offers you a drink. "Sure, I'll have a Coke," you respond.

"You want Coke or Diet Coke?" they ask, as if they don't know what they're pointing out.

Like you're supposed to respond, "Oh thanks, I don't know what I was thinking, asking for regular Coke at my size. I meant Diet Coke."

Ah, the life of an overweight American.

There are people who look down their noses at you before they meet you. Folks who make gestures when your back is turned. Short guys with "little man complex" who want to see how far they can push the gentle giant. Angry African-Americans who seize the opportunity to discriminate against the fat man the same way in which he feels discriminated against by the white man. Fire off the insults if you've got them, my friends, but you can't ask for compassion and equality if you're not willing to give it. By my early 20s I'd experienced it all and I searched even harder to understand what good could possibly come from all of this.

By 1988, tortured by my inability to put my weight problem behind me and tired of putting my future plans on hold until I was "fixed," I decided to take a negative and turn it into a positive. I began to take an interest in comedy and comedic acting. After years of using humor as a coping mechanism, I decided to try my hand at stand-up comedy. Why stand-up, you ask? Well, for one reason, the comedy boom of the late 80s was in full swing everywhere you looked. Comedy was on TV, in movies, at nightclubs, etc. Secondly, family and friends had been telling me for years that I was missing my calling as a comedian. And finally, after years of trying to find meaning in the ridiculous weight predicament I had been in, I was curious to see if I could use my "jovial" appearance and personality to my advantage. Would that not be the ultimate pay back? Take the one thing that has dogged you your entire life and make a million dollars with it. I had heard of people doing it before. Maybe, just maybe, if I could make a blessing out of a curse I'd understand why this disease was given to me. I took a night class on performing stand-up at the Boston Center For Adult Education. The course was taught by Billy Downs, one of the original owners of the Comedy Connection in downtown Boston. From there I honed my material and put together a solid seven-minute set. I tweaked the material, bounced it off a few of my friends from the radio station and signed up to perform at Open Mike Night at a local club. Ninety-nine percent of the students taking the standup comedy class had expressed nervousness over their material and their ability to try it out in an actual club. I didn't have any worries about my material. I'd been writing comedy and entertainment bits at the radio station for a couple of years by then. My worry was about how audiences and hecklers would react to jokes written by a guy who had the nerve to be fat and get up on stage. The fact that I was a big guy certainly hadn't been lost on the general public in anything else I'd ever tried to do. Would they discriminate and not laugh? Would they yell out rude comments and throw me off my game? This was the U.S.A., after all. People always have and always will look negatively at people of size.

Eventually, I convinced myself that I was simply being paranoid. Folks in the audience would have more class than that. At the end of the day humans are basically good. I still believe that. Ultimately, I convinced myself that I'd command instant respect on stage if I had the host introduce me as being from KISS 108 radio, one of the hottest stations in Boston at that time. The reality was I was as low on the totem pole as one could get. But based on the reaction from the bank tellers every week when I cashed my check, I could be the guy who cleaned the CDs and people would get excited. Just in case dropping the KISS bomb didn't command respect, I armed myself with a few fat jokes to warm up the audience should they insist I address my physical condition on stage. I also studied overweight comics like Lenny Clarke and John Pinette, two of the best in Boston, and borrowed a few anti-heckler responses should I encounter enemy fire aimed at my size. On a Wednesday night I headed into the city with my longtime friend Jimmy Harrington to the Comedy Connection on Warrenton Street for an Open Mike Showcase, hosted by comedian Jimmy Smith. When I walked into the lobby my name was in lights. Okay, I'm exaggerating here. My name was spelled out in chalk on a blackboard with eleven other open-mikers. But trust me, the dream was realized in that moment. Once the show began, I paced the back of the room and drank a couple of Pearl Harbors just to loosen up.

As my time approached I began to get nervous again, wondering if I'd get heckled during my act. "Get over yourself," I told myself repeatedly. "These people are here to laugh and support their friends." Just to give you a taste, I'll show you a transcript of the opening minutes of my set.

Jimmy Smith: "You may have heard our next act on KISS 108FM, right here in Boston. This is his first appearance. Please welcome Gary Marino!"

Me: "Thanks. Let's hear it for your host Jimmy Smith!"

Audience: (applause)

Me: "How's everybody doing tonight?"

Male Audience Member: "Fat Sh*t!"

Me: "Oh…ya…the weight. The weight I can lose. You, my friend, will always be ugly!"

Audience (laughs)

Me: "Actually, my family is pretty embarrassed about my weight. They hired the kid next door to play me in the family movies!"

Audience: (laughs)

I continued to get laughs for the rest of my set. I had some hits and I had some misses, but overall the owners of the club, as well as my friends, thought I'd done surprisingly well for my first time on stage. "You got them, held their attention and got some good laughs," one said. I went up and did a set with lesser results a few weeks later and called it quits on my comedy career right after that. Why? Well, first and foremost, stand-up just wasn't in my heart. I was, after all, trying to see if being a funny big guy could pay off. Second, I didn't realize just how strong I was for a newcomer. Unfamiliar with the art of stand-up at the time, I thought I simply didn't have it. Finally, and perhaps most importantly, I was just not comfortable getting up in front of crowds looking the way I looked. Stand-up is one of the hardest things to do in the world, and my self-confidence was pretty low as it was. It would be torture to have to get up in front of audiences every night and wonder where the next insult was coming from. Why put myself on the firing line in my vulnerable situation? Even if I were lucky enough to become successful, I knew I'd hate the way I looked in movies, on TV and on stage. Years later, when I became an agent and manager of comedians and comic actors, it occurred to me just how natural I was on stage during those two open-mike nights.

Now, did I quit because some Mr. Wonderful Schmuck decided to yell out some spineless jibberish? No, not on your life! Do I feel I would have become a strong stand-up comedian if I'd stuck with it? You bet I do. Do I have any regrets about giving up so fast? Not really. I know now that I was destined to spend the bulk of my 20s and 30s very much overweight and that would have made for an awful existence. Hating how I looked and how I felt, I'd be a Chris Farley, performing self-deprecating humor and self-parody, being tormented every time I had to watch myself on the TV screen. The more money I would have made, the more excesses I would have surrounded myself with. In time, I would have adjusted my lifestyle to my excesses. The Betty Ford Clinic. The Hazelton Rehab. It's a well known path. Eventually, after giving people a few laughs, I'd have given in to my demons. I truly believe that. The tears of a clown.

THE LIQUID DIET:
Pick a body and go with it!

By the end of 1988, liquid diets had become the rage in America. Even wildly popular talk show host Oprah Winfrey seemed to get caught up in it all. From the moment she unveiled her new body and size 8 jeans live on her program, the country was hooked on the liquid shake concept. Unfortunately for Oprah, the country also became hooked on the "Will she gain the weight back?" speculation. In the months to come, the press actually stalked Oprah at restaurants and super-markets to see if she was "off her diet again." The media sensation caught on faster then Elvis sightings. They actually filed reports about the contents on her plate.

"It appears that the glutton Oprah Winfrey has fallen off the wagon again," they wrote. "Winfrey, as seen in this exclusive photo, feasted on a 30-ounce prime rib we could only dream about. She then followed it up with a slice of cheese cake so loaded with calories that she immediately asked for a blood test. Later, Oprah stopped for fried dough and denied to the press that she was, in fact, Oprah Win-frey."

Okay, so maybe I'm exaggerating a bit here; the mainstream press wasn't that out-of-control, but the tabloids certainly were. The resulting circus-like atmo-sphere surrounding Oprah's weight only made a mockery of a very serious prob-lem in our country. It also distracted folks from her true accomplishments, which had nothing to do with her physical appearance. Her fiancée, Stedman Graham, phoned in live just to further pull on the heartstrings of people everywhere. Immediately, millions of women opened their wallets and bank accounts for the latest "Get Thin Quick" sham. And women weren't the only ones. Men like myself, who'd had enough of the slow, measured, *weigh your cottage cheese on the kitchen scale* approach, were ready to sign up for this new fast-track alternative. Liquid diet programs sprang up almost overnight at local hospitals, with actual medical professionals conducting them. These folks peddled liquid packets with names like "Optifast" and "UltraQuick." Initially, the theory seemed to make sense: drink medically safe liquid shakes 3 times per day in place of meals. Lose so much weight in the first three weeks that the results actually keep you motivated to go the rest of the distance. Not bad, at least in theory. Slow results had always chipped away at my resolve and with nearly 100 pounds to lose, I felt I was finished unless I saw instant results. Once you reached your goal weight via the liquid shakes, you would be reintroduced to healthy foods a meal at a time. First you'd add one healthy meal and cut back to two shakes. Then you would eventually phase the shakes out altogether. Radical? Maybe. But in America, we are all about the "quick fix." We all want to lose the weight, look like superstar celebrities and get back to the business of eating the foods we love as soon as possible. Unfortunately, it just doesn't work that way. Back in the winter of 1988, however, I was ready to try anything. Drastic times called for drastic measures, and I'd grown sick of looking and feeling like hell every day. I had been putting off reality for most of my life, and as college was winding down, I deeply resented the feeling that my food addiction and weight issues were holding me back from going out into the real world and shooting for my dreams. In my mind's eye, invisible bars seemed to restrain me from moving forward. Like most people, I was looking for that miracle solution, and the liquid diet programs seemed to be the answer.

Now all of these programs were charging enormous amounts of money, but you couldn't put a price on getting thin, so they were also enormously successful. I had begun to make some decent money at the radio station by then. Dipping into my savings would not be a problem either. Always on the table, of course, was the option to tap my folk's SOS (save our son) fund, so the money wasn't really a factor. I was young and figured I had my entire life to make money. This was about restarting my life with a fighting chance for success and happiness.

I signed up in the late fall for a liquid diet program that was run out of Lawrence Memorial Hospital in Medford. My Uncle Dave's fiancée at the time, Karen Howley, offered to sign up and join the program with me. She was only a couple of years older than I and had struggled with fluctuating weight throughout high school and college as well. Karen was very tall—about six feet. As a result, she never quite took the overweight thing to my level, thank God. Nevertheless, she was unhappy with herself, in the process of planning her wedding and glad to have someone to go with.

The folks running the program seemed nice enough. The group met weekly around 6:00 p.m. and weighed in with a doctor upon arrival. Blood pressures were checked and blood samples taken from each individual in the group. Then *Bang!* We were asked for a check and given our next week's supply of drink mixes. Chocolate, strawberry—or for those really missing the routine of using a utensil—a chicken soup alternative. Mmmmm! It was more like Chicken Soup Helper. After purchasing our food for the next week, we attended a sit-down class to learn about nutrition and maintenance. Of course, had the folks running the liquid program known anything about nutrition and maintenance to begin with, they'd probably not have been involved in it at all.

Within four days the weight began drastically falling off both Karen and myself. I believe I lost some ridiculous amount the first week, perhaps around 12 pounds. The shakes, although hardly anything to look forward to, seemed to hold us over. By the following week, I was already closing in on a loss of 20 pounds, with only minimal cravings for solid food. By week three I was thinking sharper and more clearly than I had in years. I actually found myself looking forward to my strawberry shakes, as well as the chicken soup alternative. I vividly remember going out to dinner with my family or friends and spooning my tasty soup, almost as if I'd ordered it off the menu. Of course the chicken soup contained no chicken, no noodles, and no vegetables. It was more like "essence of chicken soup." A lightly seasoned broth, if you can imagine. At that point it really didn't matter to me. It seemed that I was locked in for the long term on the program and ready to become a new person. That's when the trouble started. See there's one thing the folks taking your checks won't tell you about liquid diets. By week three you essentially begin freaking out and craving anything and everything. Positively anything looks good to you when you're on straight liquids for a long enough period of time. Lettuce on a stick? I'd love some! Burnt toast with hot water spread across it instead of butter? Give it to me. The houseplant in the hallway with a little Italian dressing? Well, it sure is green and leafy…The cravings were crazy and my mind began to fixate on any kind of solid food. Right around this time, my friend Michelle decided to throw a huge house party. There was a centerpiece on the table filled with fake fruit and other assorted items such as enameled raisin bread. I couldn't take my eye off the damn raisin bread. Even though I knew it was fake, it took everything I had to restrain myself. *Just let me alone with that raisin bread…oh, yeah, come over here you sweet confection…what the hell is happening to me?* In stores, I found myself sniffing scented markers (the grape-scented purple ones in particular) and buying loads of gumballs to just experience the sensation of chewing again. Ahhh, the simple pleasures in life!

In February I took the girl I'd been dating, along with her little sisters, to the New England Aquarium in Boston. Leslie was a friend of one of the disc jockeys at KISS 108. She was much younger than I was, but from the minute we met, the two of us really enjoyed each other's company. Leslie was from North Andover, MA, where she was one of eleven brothers and sisters. So on a Saturday we took some of the younger kids to see the fish at the Aquarium. When I put one of the little girls on my shoulders to view the huge 200,000-gallon tank, I was automatically dying for seafood.

"What kind of fish is that, Gary?" she asked.

"Swordfish steak," I said, smacking my lips.

"And what's that fish?" she inquired.

"Filet of sole," I sighed.

On the bottom of the massive tank, a giant, 30-lb lobster named Sam was crawling below the schools of fish. "What do they do with Sam when he dies?" asked Leslie's little sister as she sat on my shoulders. *I don't know,* I thought. *but I'm sure as hell going to find out. How about me, Sam, and a bucket of drawn butter for starters.*

The weeks without real food began to have an effect on me mentally. Although I'd lost nearly 25 pounds, I was very close to my breaking point. You see, throughout the entire time I was on just liquids, and everybody around me was eating real food. When the family was making Italian cold-cut sandwiches, I was drinking my chocolate shakes. When my friends and I ate out at Mexican or Thai restaurants, I spooned my imitation chicken soup broth, trying to ignore the hot cooked food under my nose. Folks were always supportive of my effort, but the sight of solid food wreaked havoc on my brain. Predictably, the straw that broke the camel's back came at the radio station. One evening a heavy-set man with glasses carrying a large open cardboard box walked in the door and greeted me at the front desk. I was on the phone with a listener at the time, so I motioned to the guy to hold on till I wrapped up the call. When he put the box down on the desk to wait, I noticed a half dozen white Styrofoam containers. Clearly food. The smell of the dinners (and I'm swearing on my grandmother's grave, this had nothing to do with my "food for plugs" routine) began wafting out of the box.

My senses kicked in immediately and my body suddenly came alive and began to growl. My digestive system and ketones, which had been in hibernation for the better part of a month, screamed for some real food. The delivery guy, apparently no stranger to free radio plugs, decided not to wait for me to get off the phone. As he waved good-bye he said, "These dinners are compliments of Mike's Steak house." I hung up the phone and stared at the box for the longest time. I'd been passing up free dinners for the better part of a month. My mind was transfixed by the sight and smell. My taste buds melted. I tried to think about the dangers that the coordinators of the liquid diet had warned us of. Falling off the program and shocking the body with solid food all of a sudden was strongly advised against. I knew my body would not react well to steak tips and salty fries smothered in BBQ sauce. I decided to do the right thing and leave the dinners in the FM studio for the jocks and interns to eat. The radio station was eerily quiet that night. Apparently everybody had gone home except the on-air disc jockey, a station engineer out back, and me, answering the request lines at the front desk. I took the box around the corner and down the hall to where the FM studio was. Ed McMann, the early evening jock, was busy coordinating his next hour's music and commercials when I walked in. Now he and I had shared many dinners together over the past year, but when I offered him the dinners this night, he responded, "No thanks, I'm not hungry tonight, but I'll thank them on the air." He suggested I put the dinners in the refrigerator in the cafeteria or throw them away. Not that Ed was into wasting food, but he was well aware of my liquid diet program. Hell, even he was losing weight with my "food for plugs" nonsense on hiatus.

I walked downstairs to the cafeteria with the steak tip dinners, all six sitting there, untouched, in all their glory. It was simply against my nature to not indulge, not to mention that the smell was beginning to get to me. I am only human, you know? I decided I had to have a look at the food before I placed it in the refrigerator. I took one of the containers out of the cardboard box and collapsed into a plastic chair in the café. I placed the dinner on the table and opened the cover. Classic scene: a man and his drug. Will he? Won't he? "Of all the radio joints in all the world, you had to be delivered to mine," I half joked. The glazed steak tips were sitting on top of a pile of the biggest steak fries I'd ever seen. The sight was beautiful. Pathetic of me to go on and on, I know, but trust me, they were "gorgeous," as Gram Lacam would say. I decided to look at another one of the containers, just to assure myself that the rest of the dinners were not as inviting. I lined up the second one next to the first one and took a look. This one looked even better. Giant steak tips on a mountain of warm, buttery brown rice. Nice of the folks at Mike's to offer the rice alternative instead of the fries. I glared at the dinners and tortured myself. *Could the tips be any bigger? Look at that rice. Is that Uncle Ben's?* Now I've never even liked rice, but after a month of liquid shakes, even that was beginning to torture me. I closed the tops of the containers and jammed them into the box. I vowed I would not crack under pressure. I'd already sacrificed enough, spent way too much money and been fat far too long. Just knowing that the dinners existed tortured my resolve. I surmised that if I left them in the company refrigerator they'd be eaten by the time I arrived for work the next day, but when I opened the door, a huge cake fell onto the floor. It was apparently a gift from our bakery friends in the neighboring town of Everett. One look at that jam-packed icebox, and I knew the steak tips were never going to fit. In my soul I knew I could never throw such beautiful food away, nor could I leave it to spoil on a counter somewhere. A homeless shelter would have been good, but my shift wasn't over until midnight. With my resistance slowly wearing away, I took the box into the engineer's office. "Bruce, do you want these dinners?" I asked half-heartedly. He was 5'7", maybe 160 pounds, and blessed with a normal approach to food. "No thanks. It's 8:30 p.m., too late to eat," he responded. Needless to say, at this point I was one disturbed fellow. Spiritually broken, I took the box back to the front desk. There I polished off not one, not two, but *four* of the six dinners. The steak tips were every bit as good as they looked. I attacked the steak fries mercilessly. Could somebody please cue Carly Simon's "Anticipation" please? When I awoke the next day I felt bloated and lethargic. I walked into the kitchen, grabbed the blender and my strawberry shake packet with every intention of getting back on the program. Suddenly the packets of chocolate and strawberry looked old and stale to me. I jammed them in a closet and headed for a box of cereal. Alas, the sleeping giant was awake once again.

LIFE, MARRIAGE AND
THE PURSUIT OF
EVERYTHING BUT HEALTH

Stressed Furniture-itis: An unhealthy physical disease in which severely overweight people put undo pressure on perfectly healthy furniture, causing it to violently collapse and shatter on the ground...

May 1988. A proud moment for the Salem State College Class of '88. As we filed into the gymnasium, wearing our caps and gowns, everyone in the place was on his feet applauding. The graduating class was in high spirits and reflecting positively on their achievements. Not me. I was reflecting on the fact that the chair I was sitting on was made of toothpicks and could explode at any second. As the names beginning with A's, B's, and C's were called up to receive their college degrees, I was busy strategizing on how I could keep the cheap, pathetic, Ally McBeal-sized plastic chair I was sitting on from giving out and creating a scene in front of my family and thousands of people. At first I thought about faking a medical condition. That would give me an excuse to sit somewhere else in the auditorium. Then I thought about the positions I could strike after the chair collapsed to give the illusion that it was still holding me up. We've all heard of the fetal position. Perhaps I could strike some sort of hybrid *seatal* position? *That*, I surmised, *might be tough on the knees.*

Now by all rights, the thoughts running through my head that day should have been what everyone else's were.

Four years—okay—five years of college and I finally made it. Real world, here I come. Ma and Dad haven't looked this proud since I sang "Yellow Bird" in the seventh grade concert. You know, all that stuff you think about while waiting to hear your name called to receive your degree. Of course my life was never quite that normal. I remember sitting there, planting my feet in the sumo position, putting as much pressure as I could on my legs and feet so I could buy time with the chair I was slowly killing. The actual thoughts running through my head, as I remember them, were *'Holy shit, was that a crack I just heard? Is anyone else conscious of how wobbly these things are? Okay, we're through the D's, E's and F's. If I can make it to the M's I'll grab my degree and head right for a fire exit. G's and H's. Why the hell are there so many H's? Now I know where the Jesus H. Christ comes from! I can't feel my legs anymore. I's, J's and K's. Way too long on the K's. We're not going to make it. I can feel the plastic giving way. L's and M's. Great, I've finally made it to the M's...Oh, my God! These chairs are attached to each other. If my chair collapses I could take down the rest of the M's in my row!'*

Despite my fears of causing a massive scene, the graduation ceremony finally ended without incident and I headed out to dinner with my family and Terry, another stifled would-be girlfriend.

College had been a means of ducking the real world until I could get healthy and figure out exactly what I wanted out of life. Now my college years were over and I was being forced to face the real world, ready or not. A couple of positions had opened at KISS 108, and instead of facing the discrimination that I anticipated I'd find in business world, I opted to hide out at my radio station job a couple of years longer, at least until I'd figured out how to "fix myself." Ten years after my first Weight Watchers diet, it was still all about losing the weight and figuring out who I was. In reality, the discrimination I was ducking was alive and well at KISS FM and I'd already had a taste of it. This was the look good/feel good 80s, and I was at a top ten dance station with national celebrities dropping by every day. From a looks perspective, I probably should have been across town somewhere at a classic rock station. There were plenty of guys like me over there, but I was curious to see if a career at KISS could pan out for me. One person on my side was station boss Sunny Joe White, one of the founders of the station. Sunny had incredible compassion for people and their problems. He was no different with me. He always had a way of letting me know that I needed to get healthy in order to be in the running for anything tangible at the station, but he never seemed to lose hope that someday I would. From time to time over the years, Sunny even bumped into my mom at a mall somewhere and he always inquired if I was trying to lose weight. Whether I liked it or not, my life was always tied to my size. I went on to work another two years at KISS FM, doing everything from answering phone calls at the front desk to writing and producing on-air bits and recording jingles and song spoofs. To pick up extra money I worked security for celebrity guests and announced news and weather on KISS' sister station, WXKS-AM. Every once in awhile on the FM side I even got asked to co-host a radio shift and be an on-air sidekick. Like most broadcasting companies, KISS had its share of tough individuals, but it also had some gentle, non-judgmental people. With the exception of one of the nighttime jocks and myself, no one else was over-weight.

By the end of 1988, the morning show host had been asking for guys to work security out in the lobby because of all of the celebrity guests coming in for his show. Earlier that year, when Patrick Swayze dropped by, close to 300 fans stormed the parking lot. A bunch of us who had been working as part-timers signed up. In retrospect, that was a big mistake. The place already had a low opinion of me because of my appearance. Now I was the gorilla in charge of securing the building and checking in celebrities. They seemed to develop selec-tive amnesia when it came to the creative work I'd done at the station for nearly three years. All the while, my locker swelled with dozens upon dozens of air-check tapes and pre-recorded bits I had produced. I was pretty much at the bot-tom of the totem pole, working three part-time positions to round out a forty-plus hour workweek. I also made my share of mistakes, learning as any 23-year-old does along the way.

Despite my perceived shortcomings, terrific memories and lasting friendships were born out of my KISS experience. One Monday morning in September, 1989, I opened the Boston Globe on my lunch break and noticed a full-page ad: "Jenny Craig Weight Loss Centers comes to Boston." The company had begun a massive publicity campaign in the Boston area. Desperate to rid myself of my food addiction and have some forward motion in my life, I joined up that evening. For the sake of sparing you another failed diet story, I'll cut right to the vital statistics:

- Roughly $70.00 or so per week for frozen dinners and "Jenny Bars" (snack bars)
- 35-pound weight loss in 8 weeks before cracking from the pressure of my "Food Plan"
- Dated two of the sweetest and most helpful weight loss counselors I've ever met in my life (introduced my friends to their friends and had some terrific times)

By late October, the Jenny Craig Weight Loss Plan had joined the growing list of failed diets in my life. Problem was, I still had about 40 of those "Jenny Bars" in my refrigerator at home. How does one get rid of them? The way anyone one does when you're off the wagon: Jenny Bar with Captain Crunch for breakfast. Two Jenny Bars in the car on the way to work. Another one with the Big Mac and fries at lunch and another 3 to 4 in the movie theater that night (along with a $12 box of Klondikes and a ridiculous-sized hot buttered popcorn).

Meanwhile, back at KISS FM, despite looking like a fish out of water, there were occasionally times when the higher-ups would overlook my sloppy physical condition enough to compliment me on my on-air work. "Hey, Big Guy, I liked that jingle you recorded the other day for the nighttime show." Or "If you want to do some stuff on my show tomorrow, let me know." Even with the compliments, my instinct was that I was viewed as a lost cause who had no real respect for himself. In December of 1989, massive layoffs across the board put an abrupt end to my attempt at a radio career. The recession had begun and the firing of over 20 people was immediate. The station was trimming the, er, *fat*. I was fine with the pink slip. Fresh out of college, I'd had my share of hits and misses at KISS. By then I was nearly 24 years old, 324 pounds, burned out, and sick of my food-for-plugs nonsense. Thanks to a generous offer from my Uncle Dave, I headed off to his place on Marco Island, Florida to rejuvenate myself. It was time to move on, but before I could do that I was bound and determined to end my life-long battle with overeating.

In southwest Florida, better known as "Heaven's Waiting Room," I hit the ground running. Walking the beach every morning, playing tennis in the afternoons and swimming whenever I had the chance. In February of 1990 I had a brief relationship with a girl named Maria, from the city of Golden Gate. Maria was a living doll with long brown hair, gorgeous blue eyes, a gentle soul and a curious spirit, the likes of which I have never encountered since. On weekends, when Maria wasn't working, we'd rent a Boston Whaler and head out to the mini-islands off the coast of Marco and The Isle of Capri. All things considered, it was a surreal time in my life and I felt as if I was on some kind of radio producer relocation program. As we lay on the white sand in the south Florida sunshine, I would joke with Maria, "The water's warm, the drinks are cold, and I don't know the names of the disc jockeys." Returning to the mainland, it never took long to realize that Maria and I were from two very different worlds. Eventually it ended for all the right reasons, but let's face it, even when you know in your heart it's not right, it still hurts like hell to let go and move on. The exercise, combined with the broken-heart diet, resulted in some substantial weight loss. I guess you could say I was gaining on the problem again.

A guy can't be on vacation forever, and by early April I returned home with renewed optimism and hope. The economy in Massachusetts was in complete disarray when I returned. Companies were undergoing massive layoffs and closing their doors to all new applicants. At 250 pounds, I was leaner, meaner and sporting a college degree, but the recession was severe and it was obvious that I'd be needing a lot more than physical health and a degree to land a career job. I visited my old boss Sunny Joe to show him I had pulled it somewhat together and he quickly offered me a freelance writing and production job. "I liked those jingles and promos you did last year," he said. It was nice confirmation that at least someone had recognized the good work I'd done, but I politely declined, feeling it was truly time to try something new.

Right around this time my Uncle David mentioned that he could use me part-time in his Boston office, organizing and categorizing his company's video library. I'd been very close to him from the time I was 6 or 7 years old and I relished the opportunity to be around him. Lordly and Dame, Inc. had been around since the 1950s, and by the 70s was one of Boston's most active entertainment and speaker agencies. My uncle explained to me that his company was now using VHS videotapes to sell acts and he needed a solid system in place to do so. I may have been slightly over-qualified for the job, but I jumped at the chance to see how another business operated and made money. Among the legions of nine-to-fivers, I was on the 7:45 a.m. train to the city every day. The experience was new and refreshing and the 40-minute walks from the train station to the office were good for my body, which was beginning to show signs of regaining some of the weight I'd lost in Florida. On my first day in the office I was immediately intrigued when my uncle showed me his company's collection of marketing videos. I had no idea that videotapes were that widely used. There were stacks, piles, shelves and boxes full of VHS tapes of comedians, magicians, and national recording acts. Every motivational speaker, novelty act and musician seemed to be selling themselves with videotapes. The days of an entertainer getting work from a head shot and a resumé were apparently long over. From that point on, I knew there was a niche in producing videos for performers.

On my first day at Lordly & Dame I met Julie Harmon, the office manager. She was sweet, beautiful, and mysterious. From the moment I set eyes on her, I was filled with this mind-blowing feeling that she would one day be a very big part of my life. I wasn't sure exactly what part; maybe she'd become an important friend. Perhaps a business partner. Maybe a wife. Possibly all three. I just wasn't sure. The feeling was unlike any other I'd had in my life. Then again, I could count the meaningful female relationships I'd had on one hand. Now, even with all the chemistry in the room that day, it would take me another 6 months of working together to actually have a conversation and get to the first date with Julie Harmon. Why? Well, I could read books. I could read facial expressions. I could read body language. Heck, I could even read a little Braille here and there. But to this day, reading women is a skill I've yet to master. It took me half a year to understand that when a woman shows no interest, walks out of the room every time you enter and refuses to even make eye contact, it means that she is, in fact, genuinely interested. Obviously. Who knew? So on a January day in 1991 I finally figured it out and asked Julie on a date. We were joined at the hip from that day on. Ahhh, young love! Breakfast at her place. Lunch at the mall food court. Dinner and drinks at the Mexican Cantina down the street. And just to top it off, ice cream on the way home. You can hear the music now, can't you? That's Herman's Hermits, "Something tells me I'm into something good," you hear. And she's playfully flirting with me on the way into her apartment while I'm playing the Leslie Nielsen part and knocking over potted plants and missing half of what she's saying at any given time.

By the time we got engaged, 10 months later, I'd gained more than 70 pounds. Once again I looked out of shape and felt horrible. Miraculously, It seemed to make no difference to Julie at all. I was baffled and mystified by her tolerance. For years I'd seen relationships go south because of my looks and the inability to stabilize my health. Most ended with the words "Maybe down the line, if you get your act together…" Now a woman, and a beautiful one at that, didn't seem to care. In a world where everyone is judged unfairly by looks, I found someone who went with what she saw inside. Maybe love was blind or Julie was simply cut from a different cloth. I didn't care. I gave that girl a ring.

Once we got engaged that October, I decided I needed to do two things before the wedding day. First was the obligatory *lose the weight* so I could look good in the wedding photos. Who wants their kids looking at the wedding album someday and seeing a John Candy look-alike groom? The second thing I needed to do was get an actual career job. Well, as the saying goes, one out of two ain't bad.

Which one do you think I delivered on?

During our annual trek to New York City each December my friends and I met up with an old school acquaintance named Lisa Fina. We'd gone to school together back in the St. Joseph's days. At the time she was working in the wardrobe department at Radio City Music Hall. One night Lisa mentioned that she'd just designed a dress for Neicey Boswell, a singer from back home who performed regularly at The Roxy Club in Boston. "Her manager is looking for someone to produce a video to send to record labels. Can you do that?" she asked. I joked that after nearly a year and a half without steady work I could do just about anything. I took down the manager's number—a man named Richard Wolfson—and had the job even before I arrived home from New York. A few Saturdays later I borrowed a camera, shot the video at The Roxy, edited it at my alma mater Salem State and presented it to him a week later. Receiving that first check was empowering and, frankly, helpful in paying off the credit card companies who were stalking me at that point. I decided to head out on that highway known as self-employment and I never looked back. I created a company that specifically produced videos for entertainers to market their talents. Between 1992 and 1995 I produced videos for standup comedians, theater groups, television and film actors, stage hypnotists, rock & roll bands, speakers, and pretty much anyone who could write my name on a check. Actually it wasn't my name at all they were writing on the checks. It was "GAMA Video." Early on I'd been stuck for a name to call my production company, so I asked my Uncle Dave what he thought if I just abbreviated my name using the first two letters of my first and last name. Unoriginal you might say? He didn't like it either, but I went with it anyway.

Building GAMA Video was one of the most invigorating experiences I've ever had. Growing up and coming of age with a serious weight problem, I had been delaying reality and dealing with life reactively for most of my teens and 20s—key years, people will tell you. But now I was taking action to build my future and I wasn't about to let my weight problem get in the way. I started the company from scratch: no backers, no equipment, no small business loans and less than $2000 in the bank. The recession of the early 1990s had hit Massachusetts hard and the words "budget cuts" were all over the place. Yet slowly, I was adding clients, equipment and freelance production people to my team. Julie was handling contracts and administrative details. Within a period of 18 months, GAMA had gone from a part-time job to a full-time endeavor. What a country! Unfortunately, with business success came personal failure. Working nonstop had taken a toll on my weight. I was sedentary for months on end and was clearly pinching 300 pounds again. I was 27 years old, and feeling 60. Right around that time in my life I began to lose my desperate passion to get thin. Too many years of living on a roller coaster ride, waiting to see if I could lose the weight, had taken a toll on my psyche. I'd grown tired of putting off plans my entire life. By this time I had spent well over a decade battling the bulge, desperately trying to fix myself with every new scam diet out there. Every TV pitchman who proclaimed "The only thing you have to lose is the weight," every liquid diet operating out of some hospital back room, every revolutionary herbal treatment. It had all just pushed me too far. I decided that I had given it everything I had and it was time to move on. I studied people in my life who had become very successful in spite of their weight problems. People like my uncle, who owned his own business, three homes and a 40-foot boat. He was married, about to become a father, and appeared to love his life. I'd never seen anyone insult him, hassle him or approach him about his weight. Yet with me it was always front and center. "The Unc," as we called him, had a great sense of humor and always seemed to be remarkably unaffected by his weight problem. He was an inspiration to me early on because he'd been able to put together a prosperous life. Could I create a similar existence? I was sure as hell going to try! I looked at folks like Diana Steele, one of the disc jockeys I'd worked with during my radio years at KISS 108FM. She'd managed to become a major market on-air personality who was making plenty of money. Diana was also in demand making paid personal appearances. "Lady D" always seemed to have a lot of toys around, too. New cars, trendy pets and attractive love interests that rivaled anything you'd see in Hollywood. I decided that if those people could achieve success without losing the weight, I could too. GAMA Video would be my ticket. I was young, about to be married, and creatively on fire. Cosmetic issues were what high-schoolers stressed out about. I was heading for big places, unfortunately on many levels.

As our wedding day approached in the spring of 1993, I rushed to take care of whatever details needed to be handled. I was resigned to the fact that on the biggest day of my life, the one where you want to look your best, I'd be taking it to the aisle the biggest I'd ever been. Plenty of other engaged folks had lost that battle and I simply made peace with it. Undaunted, we went on to have a spirited and wonderful wedding. On May 15th, 1993, the sun was shining, the warm winds were blowing, and in Julie's hometown of Westfield, Massachusetts, the two of us tied the knot. At our reception we sang, danced, and got downright silly with over 150 guests. The day was perfect, tight tuxedo and all.

On our honeymoon, in Marco Island, Florida, always one of my favorite vacation spots, things were perfect as well. Then about 6 days into the honeymoon, after swimming, relaxing and exploring, Julie and I decided to check out the nightlife in southwest Florida. There really wasn't much at the time in terms of clubs, and when we arrived at Septembers Night Club, we chuckled at the sign on the door: "Comedy Night Tonight." At home with GAMA Video, I'd been spending 2-3 nights per week in comedy clubs in Boston. I'd cut deals with many of the clubs to be their exclusive in-house production company. Now, on our honeymoon, on the one night we decided to go out, the only real nightclub on the entire island was throwing a stand-up comedy night. We laughed and bought two tickets. I was sitting several rows back that night, wearing my loudest flowered shirt, drinking Piña Coladas with Julie, when the first comic—a young man named Alex P. Ferret (not his real name, but trust me you've never heard of him)—took to the stage. Alex was a young, smart-aleck type who had all the right ingredients except the most important one: being funny. By the time his first half dozen or so jokes crashed and burned, Alex P. did what most desperate comics do and turned on the audience to get laughs. "Hey, you in the flowered shirt," he baited me. "The guy all wrapped up in the health thing. What's your story?". *Okay here it comes,* I remember thinking. *Can't a guy just enjoy his honeymoon with his new wife without some punk comic mouthing off?* A few more cheap insults aimed at my size came my way and as I sat there, I began to get agitated. Alex P. went on to, as they say in the comedy business, "eat it" for another 15 minutes or so. When he finally stomped off the stage, girl scout style, at the end of his performance (performance might be an overstatement) he walked right past me, trying hard not to make eye contact. As pissed off and embarrassed as I was, something told me to let it go, because at some point down the line our paths would cross. My intuition has always been one of my better senses.

Two years later, Alex P. Ferret began sending promo tapes to corporate and club agents all over Boston. I personally saw to it that his videotapes were recycled and given to club owners' wives to tape "Melrose Place" with. A few years after that, the inevitable call came to my office from Alex himself to see if I could help him "break into the Boston scene." Let's just say Alex P. learned a thing or two about insulting his audience members. *You never know who's sitting there, so watch who you use as fodder, pal.* Last time I checked, Alex P. Ferret had yet to break into the Boston scene, or come to think of it, any scene at all. If you're keeping score, that's Big guys 2, wise guy Comedian 0.

By 1995 GAMA Video was housing New England's largest library of performer videos. My company was making solid money, thanks to strategic partnerships with people like Scott Horgan, a whiz kid at sound, lighting and production support, and guys like Paul DiPanfilo, who could produce CDs, DVDs and promotional marketing tools that were second to none. I rented work space in

Burlington, MA and hired an office assistant. I brought a CPA into the office every Friday to handle the books. I found the best camera people I could and had the ability to put together teams for each individual project. As the company developed into a junior-packaging company, I kept involving Julie in everything I could, from marketing and creative decisions to administrative and technology issues.

As the business grew, the restaurant menu folder in my receptionist's desk began growing as well. At the office, not a day went by that we didn't order pizzas, Chinese food or specialty sandwiches. It was the same old Gary, only with a new set of food-loving friends to eat with. At night I'd be out at restaurants, trying to close deals with clients, or at events where the buffets never seemed to stop. The company revenues were growing, but so was my waistline and already stressed physical condition. Ignoring my imperfect health to build the perfect company was a flawed approach, to say the least. The only one who didn't seem to notice was me.

My health wasn't the only thing I was ignoring. Parenthood, or the act of being responsible for someone besides yourself, went on the backburner in a big way. Basically because, well, I was in a big way. As I've already explained, delaying reality is a symptom of being an overweight food addict, and this extended to the concept of having children with Julie. Philosophically speaking, we'd been married fairly young by today's standards. We were around 27 years old, so becoming parents wasn't exactly the first thing on our agenda. But as 29 becomes 30, and then suddenly 32, the natural stage is to gravitate to starting a family. Seemingly everywhere Julie and I went, people were all over us about the kid thing.

"When are you two gonna have a little one?"

"What are you waiting for?"

My answer would always be the same.

"I'm not convinced I should be reproduced at this point," I'd say.

I'd joke with people, but behind the joking were some very serious feelings. Why should I have a little version of myself when this version had some serious defects to be worked out? I honestly couldn't even fathom the idea of becoming a father. For those that think I'm exaggerating my addiction here, perhaps creating a mountain out of a molehill, feel free to skip ahead to the chapter on Sleep Apnea. Then take two aspirin and phone your therapist in the morning.

Now I love children, and I think becoming a dad is one of the greatest experiences a guy can have. I've spent more time being an uncle to my nieces and nephew than a lot of folks do, but the truth is I really never wanted to have kids until I "fixed" my longtime addiction and weight problem. I simply never believed that a person my size could properly parent. Now you don't need to be an Olympic athlete, but at the same time, when the little one in diapers has lost his balance and is heading for the floor, you do need to be able to run and be their landing pad, don't you? Being a parent means having a good deal of energy, but I was physically exhausted by 11 in the morning, so I put it on the back burner and concentrated on what was on the front burner: food, lots and lots of food.

MEET MR. PIVOT:
Sports and Weight Gain

By the time I met my wife, married and started my company, I wasn't into playing sports or exercising very much. People around me could never seem to understand the lack of any physical activity in my life. The truth was, I'd never developed into a strong athlete as a kid, and therefore had no interest in pursuing anything athletic now either. To me, staying away from the tennis courts and ball fields was a positive thing, because whenever I entered the game there were simply no winners or losers. *Everybody lost.* Thanks to my boyhood football coach, the Bulldog, strenuous exercise was not my favorite thing to do. To put it bluntly, I'd never learned the meaning of "it hurts so good."

Making matters worse was my physical condition, which only hampered my ability to do just about anything athletic. In my opinion, being overweight affects different people in different ways. In my case, the weight made me mentally exhausted on the playing field.

In high school, my sophomore and junior years on the lacrosse field were a testament to this. Since I wasn't a fast runner, middle and attack positions were out of the question. Due to my size, defense made the most sense. The problem was that I became mentally fatigued during the action. I was not exactly the most spry player anyone had ever seen. By the time I noticed the guy running at our goal with the ball, I had already let him into my territory and he'd wind up to take his shot. I would then snap awake so fast I'd virtually attack him with my Lacrosse stick. One off the helmet! Penalty. Two to the facemask! Two more infractions. Here's another one to the collarbone! Who's counting any more? Boom! There's the whistle. Penalty on Marino. Thanks, ref, I was ready for a rest. I was sidelined for the rest of the game.

There was one thing I was good at during Lacrosse season; that was raising money for uniforms, equipment and transportation. As with most high schools at the time, the individual team members would be asked to raise money by selling

M&M's. Each of us would be given a case containing 100 boxes or so. I, of course, knew I would eat my entire case, plain and peanut. These folks had just given heroin to an addict. *Who do I make the check out to for my case, coach?*

At the age of 19 I took up the game of golf. It seemed like a game that could be friendly to the big & tall man. You rode around in a cart, wearing sunglasses and a loud pastel shirt and clobbered the ball as it sat innocently on the tee. I developed my signature slice to the right-hand side of the fairway almost instantly. Like most golfers, I blamed it on bad habits, clubs that needed to be re-gripped, my need for a private trainer and of course my ever present weight problem. "You need your weight evenly distributed on your body when you follow through with your swing," was one trainer's advice. I remember thinking, *Sir, if I could redistribute this weight around my body as I saw fit, I wouldn't be hanging out talking with a bunch of guys in pleated pants, now would I?*

Next up was the game of tennis. How hard could it be? Heck, I was only about 10, 20, 30, perhaps 110 pounds overweight at that point. I purchased a top-of-the-line Prince tennis racket, an instructional video by Bjorn Borg and a pair of size 12 tennis shoes. Little Gary was combat ready. First up, I challenged my friend Jimmy Harrington's mother (70 years old at the time) to a match. Maybe it was my weight, maybe it was my ADD, maybe she was a phenomenal tennis player for a woman her age. Needless to say, Mrs. H showed me a thing or two. In 1990 I joined the Winchester Indoor Tennis Club and kept it to strictly playing with family members. Eventually I earned the name "Mr. Pivot" from playing tennis, meaning I'd pivot left to hit the ball, I'd pivot right to hit the ball, but I wasn't ever gonna go running for that ball. I wasn't in any shape to be trying any of that running stuff. Not at my weight.

Even sports such as skiing seemed impossible once I found myself on the other side of 250 pounds. A girlfriend named Maureen once talked me into going to a ski resort in Vermont. Now there wasn't much out there for the big guys, in terms of ski outfits and accessories. So there I was, heading out on the slopes dressed like a landscaper in July. Immediately I felt awkward in the ski getup, and my 6E-width feet could barely fit into the ski boots. "Let's do the black diamond slope. You're good enough!" said Maureen.

I closed my eyes and invited complete denial onto my brain. "Sure, I think I can handle it," I responded. As the two of us rode a ski lift that seemed to disappear into the clouds, it dawned on me that I hadn't seen any other folks like me (people of size) anywhere else on the slopes. I wished I'd joined them that day. When we got to the top of the mountain, I dismounted the lift awkwardly. My feet were numb from the ski boots that didn't fit and my weight was distributed unevenly on my body. To put it bluntly, I was in heavy people's hell. Okay, first problem: right out of the gate I crashed when we had to exit the ski lift. When I got up, my pants were lower than a plumber could have ever imagined. Half of my butt was exposed and filled with snow. As I headed down the mountain, I immediately realized that there was too much weight on my knees and back to properly ski. I wiped out roughly every thirty seconds. Eventually, with Maureen long gone, I decided to end my misery, take my chances and ski straight down the mountain. Go for broke! As I approached the bottom of the hill, going way too fast, I noticed an unfortunate detail: a ski class directly in my way. Somehow I collapsed onto my back in an attempt to wipe out before I crashed into the entire group, but my skis remained flat on the ground while I lay flat on my back, the whole time going at a good clip. Got the visual? I crashed through the middle of the entire class, all on my back. All I can remember is seeing hats, poles, and skiing apparatus flying everywhere in my wake. My fall was eventually broken by none other than the windows of the ski lodge. When I walked into the lodge bar to find Maureen ten minutes later, the place broke out into actual applause. I decided I'd stick with snowmobiles from that point on.

BUILDING SOMETHING
BESIDES A SANDWICH

In the American lexicon, "producer" is an overused word. You can produce a talent show or a submarine sandwich these days and call yourself a producer. I'm very skilled at both. Producing performer marketing tapes may have been how my company started, but at GAMA we were being asked to do a lot of different things. A creative blend of casting, talent consulting, artist management and booking, special event production, treatment writing and, of course, video production, was going on. By mid-1995 I had changed the company's name to Harmon-Marino Entertainment and we began taking the process to the next natural step: booking and managing the talents we had on tape for the corporate, special event and casting markets. I'd designed the company after the talent management and production companies I'd read about in New York and Los Angeles. Those companies managed a stable of talent and produced their own projects as well. There were no companies doing that in Boston, and I figured Harmon-Marino had a chance to be a real player someday. By 1998, as a result of Julie's and my hard work, Harmon-Marino was blossoming into a unique entertainment company. We had the ability to package writers, actors, comedians, music acts, directors and behind-the-scenes people for customized live shows or entertaining videos. I commenced working with creative writers like Michael Coleman and talented up and coming comics like Matty Blake, Tom Briscoe and John Turco. I also began working with seasoned comic actors like Tony V., who'd made national appearances in shows like "Seinfeld" and "Late Night with Conan O'Brien" and musical acts like Mark Morris and Catunes. I formed a strategic alliance with George Tobia, an entertainment attorney who represented talents like Kiefer Sutherland, Richard Lewis, Hunter S. Thompson, and Hollywood producers like Andre Barnwell. I wasn't becoming rich, but I'd achieved a certain degree of success producing projects and performing artists, all the while being my own boss. I was making a living by being creative. No one could judge me or hold my job over my head because of my appearance. I was, at last, my own island.

Building the company from the ground up was one of the most satisfying accomplishments in my life. In 1998, with the help of my friend and client Vinnie Sestito, the talent management end of my business began to blossom as well.

That's where the old common denominator—the weight problem—came back into play. As an agent or manager of actors, musicians or standup comedians, you spend countless hours designing and tweaking your artist's image. You help craft everything from their looks to their material to their promotional videos and press kits. It may be the talent that has the magic on stage, but you have to sell the artist's image to get them on stage to begin with.

By 2000, in the process of dissecting and scrutinizing other people's images, I began to take a look at my own. What I saw, I did not like. At 35, I was the quintessential picture of bad health. Tight fitting, style-less clothes gripped my body. Dark circles under my eyes seemed to be in place constantly. My brain was seemingly overdosed by details at all times and my bloated, sloppy appearance gave the impression of a man spending way too much time building his career and not enough time looking in the mirror. Jean shirts, sweat pants and baseball caps with extra-long brims flipped on my head and worn backwards made the "urban camouflage" look from my high school years actually seem stylish. *Ladies, don't let this one get away!*

In hindsight, what good was building an entertainment dynasty if I would never live to enjoy it? And if I did live, all the money in the world wouldn't change the "no quality of life" status I was living with. I had high hopes for Harmon-Marino (H/M), but as time went on, it became apparent that the company wasn't growing in size. It was grossing impressive numbers, but the net was, well, somewhat gross. H/M always felt bigger because of the freelance and part-time help, but the money just never seemed to be there to hire more people. The steps that were required to provoke the company to grow into a bona fide success could not be carried out by a person who was out of shape and mentally drained. Now every person out there is different, and some people may have been able to take H/M to the next level, regardless of their health. But as I've pointed out all along, for me the food addiction and weight gain seemed to S.C.U.D. missile my ability to be a player in the business world. Despite my company's ability to keep busy through recessions, terror attacks and everything else, I was simply not running a good operation. I had neither the stamina, energy level, nor physical ability to turn H/M into a talent agency and production company with many employees and big-paying clients.

I've tried to emphasize all along that for me, obesity and food issues were a real monster. Not everybody is affected both physically and mentally. Although major opportunities occasionally came my way, I never felt up to the challenge in the shape I was in. In 1998 a hot new management company in Los Angeles was interested in having Harmon-Marino operate as an East Coast wing of their company. A meeting in Hollywood was proposed. To win these folks over I knew I'd need a certain degree of polish, but my confidence lagged. I had been to Los Angeles a couple of times, but now we were talking about a big meeting with some serious players. Hollywood was truly the land of the fit and beautiful. Nowhere else in the world did looks count like they did there.

I could not gather up the confidence to make the live pitch or even book the flight. As a result, the trail went cold. This scenario was nothing new. Thus taking my small company to the next level, in terms of size and profit margin, was going to be tough, so I decided to rethink my previous strategy. I needed to build a successful human first, then a successful company. Although H/M had generated a good deal of money for a lot of people over the years, the problem that was holding me back then, and that had held me back my entire life, was still consuming me.

BLESSED WITH GOOD TEETH

By the time I was in my 30s I was keenly aware that furniture—name brand or not—was not exactly a friend to the "men of girth." I'd crashed my share of chaise lounges, bar stools, wooden bed frames and deck chairs over the years. Out of embarrassment, I'd at times quickly make myself scarce before anybody ever noticed. Sometimes I'd leave cash to pay for the damage. One chair I never had to pay for and always felt secure about was the good old traditional dentist's chair. Heavy folks will know what I'm referring to here. Dentists' chairs are so solid you'd think NASA made them, right? One afternoon in 1995, during a routine checkup, our longtime family dentist, Dr. Philip Richardson, finished his examination, put his dental tools down and nodded his head approvingly. "Mr. Marino, you have been blessed with good teeth," he said. Now I had to laugh at that one. Here I was, 376 pounds, but I'd been "blessed" because my teeth were stellar.

"Doc, let's be frank," I quickly responded. "I'd trade these for a pair of Austin Powers molars in a second if I could just trim 100 pounds off myself."

Dr. Richardson laughed. "Just be grateful for what you have; those are healthy teeth," he responded. Of course he wasn't the only doctor to tell me that I should be grateful for my health.

A few years earlier another doctor, this one from Massachusetts General Hospital, had echoed the same sentiments. "Mr. Marino," he said. "I'd like to get angry with you over your escalating weight problem, but your last set of test results are in, and the bottom line is your cholesterol is perfect and your blood pressure is better than mine."

Another doctor at Mass General, a sports medicine specialist, told me that my body was remarkably unaffected by all my years of being overweight. No back problems, no knee problems, not even a hernia for my trouble. Not bad when you think about it. In fact, for years people I came into contact with had been confessing to me that they were amazed at my fast pace and spry ability to get around. The reality was, however, that their opinions of me were always pretty low to begin with. Thin people always seemed to automatically size me up as a dead man walking, even though sometimes they were the ones with blood pressure monitors strapped to themselves. That's America for you. We all judge the person next to us without ever looking in the mirror first. Then again, looks can be deceiving at times.

My cousin Eddie was 6'2", 45 years old, a lifelong runner and the proverbial picture of health. Sometime around 1996, Eddie stayed with my wife and me a few days a week during a cushy consulting gig in Boston. One summer night, around 10 p.m., I arrived home from work and decided to finish up the previous night's leftovers. The key word here being "summer," because that meant that the leftovers would be steaks and grilled potatoes from the nightly barbecue the previous evening. Ahhh, there's nothing like putting a 20-ounce London broil smothered in BBQ sauce in your gut at 10 p.m., right? By the way, the potatoes were also smothered in—you guessed it—BBQ sauce. Eddie walked through the door, looked at the platter of food I was eating and shrewdly kept his thoughts to himself. *This guy's over the top* was probably one of them. Eddie decided to join me for a bite, but not what I was having. He headed for the refrigerator and grabbed his "special" bran muffins. You know the muffins, the ones that are high-fiber, low-calorie, no-fat and extremely lacking in taste for people with dangerously high cholesterol. When he sat down on the other side of the table, the two of us began laughing hysterically at the ridiculous nature of the situation. The 370-pound guy in the Hawaiian shirt was eating the super-sized steak and potato platter. The svelte 170-pound guy in the running suit was eating a special bran muffin to control his dangerously high cholesterol. What a TV commercial that scene would have made! "Why is the man on the left smiling?" the voice announcer would have asked. The ironic part was that we both should have been eating each other's meals. It occurred to me not long after that night just how lucky I'd been up until that point in my life. Years and years of gorging myself and packing on the pounds and still no Type #2 diabetes, no blood pressure problems, no cholesterol issues or back problems. However, life has a funny way of making things change just when you finally have learned to appreciate what you have. Just when I thought I had dodged the health bullet, my luck was about to run out.

SLEEP APNEA: WAKE UP ALREADY!

I woke up one September morning in the fall of 1996 feeling dizzy and exhausted. Not completely uncommon for a guy who drank beer and ate like a king, but on this particular morning there was something different. I sat on the edge of the bed for what seemed like forever, trying to tune in to the queasy feeling I had in my head. It was unlike anything I had ever felt, almost like I'd somehow sleepwalked my way to a brutal third shift job in the early morning hours, worked my tail off and returned to my bed 20 minutes before my alarm clock went off. A faint, white-colored froth encircled my mouth, which was as disturbing as the dizziness I was experiencing. *What the hell happened to me last night?* I thought. Later, I showered and drove to my office. However, the lack of equilibrium did not go away, and I began to wonder if it was more than an exceptionally bad night of sleep. My suspicions were confirmed the very next day when I awoke with the same feeling and once again, a faint white paste surrounded my mouth. *What is going on with me?* I may have been over 370 pounds to my friends, but I was impeccable about my hygiene issues. Drooling while I slept was simply unacceptable. By the third day I arose with the feeling that something was deeply wrong with me, but once again I ignored it and got on with the day. My company was taping an interview that morning with nationally acclaimed Chef Robert Cardoos. On the way home from the video shoot, my cameraman was driving and mentioned that I had seemed low-key during the interview. I responded that I was fine and asked him how he thought the shoot had gone. As he was answering my question, I faded off into an exhausted sleep. Either his answer was exceptionally boring or there was something seriously wrong with me. By the fourth night of quasi sleep I was increasingly disturbed by my inability to rest properly. It's like anything else in life, you just don't realize what you have until it's gone. Talk to anyone who's ever developed a sleep disorder and you'll realize just how precious a solid night's sleep is.

As the weeks slowly passed by, a new addition to my sleep dysfunction was brought to my attention by my wife and anyone else who had been an audience to my constant napping routine. Apparently loud snoring and snorting sandwiched long periods of time when my breathing seemed to stop. As the autumn of 1996 dragged on, I began a daily ritual of napping in the early afternoon. Heck, I even sprang for a brand new leather couch for my office. You know the one, black with layers of puffy cushioning. When they were meeting with clients, the guys in my office would occasionally use my computer's fish tank screen saver (the one with the aquarium sound effects) to drown out my snoring. That was one way to deal with it, I guess. I remember the draining, helpless feeling of hearing my phone ring during these naps and not having the capacity to snap out of my coma-like state. There was something different about these types of naps. I had no control over when they started and when they stopped. An eerie fatigue would slowly come over my body, and when it did, I was paralyzed, usually with just enough time to find a place to lie down.

Early on, when the symptoms began to appear, my mom began to stress out. Unfortunately, I'd fallen asleep in her presence more than a few times, segueing into my snore-and-snort show. Throw in a routine where you stop breathing and you've got every parent's nightmare. One day in December of 1996, Ma walked into my office with a "Dear Abby" article. The woman in the article had just lost her 31-year-old son (same age as me) to a sleep disorder named Obstructive Sleep Apnea. The symptoms were exactly like mine—a Xerox copy of what I'd been experiencing. I tried hard not to let my mother know how much the article hit home. The story described how the disease affects overweight people when they sleep. Apparently the neck and throat muscles relax whenever the mind reaches the deep sleep stage, blocking the windpipe. For the affected, this occurs dozens of times per night, causing the heart to race with every cycle. No REM stage for these people; they simply stopped breathing and awakened only when they were choking for air. Frightening! The woman who wrote the article wanted Dear Abby to reprint the story so that other mothers would take action with their kids if they had these symptoms. "I'm terrified I'll lose you to this, Gary. Terrified," said Rainbow. Of course by this time these conversations were old hat between us. Nevertheless, the Dear Abby article hit home. On my mother's request, I signed up for a sleep study in January of 1997.

The sleep study took place at Massachusetts General Hospital and involved a specialist putting electrodes all over my body and videotaping my entire night's sleep. The results intimated that I had a mild-to-strong case of Sleep Apnea. *Con-*

grats, I remember thinking to myself. *You're the stuff Dear Abby articles are made of.* I'd somehow eaten myself into some type of bizarre sleeping disease. The question now was what was I to do about it? My productivity at work was dropping off considerably. Dark circles around my eyes had become part of my daily look. I began loading up my secretary, Lucy Mathews, with things to do in the mornings while I slept on my couch during the long afternoons. I then put in my office work after hours, during the night, or on weekends, whenever I could muster up the energy. My life began to feel like a light that was fading fast, and there I slept, powerless to do anything about it.

The solution to this problem was, of course, simple. Lose the weight. But since it was clear that I wasn't any closer to doing that, I was prescribed C-PAP Therapy.

"C-PAP Therapy?" I asked my doctor.

"Gary, your condition is serious. This is nothing to play games with. Until you lose 150 pounds or better you'll have to sleep with a machine called a C-PAP. It stands for Continuous Positive Airway Pressure. You'll wear a full facemask with a tube attached to this machine. The specialists who conducted your sleep study strongly recommend it."

I listened in horror as my doctor described how the flow of air provided by the C-PAP would keep the muscles in my throat from collapsing so I could sleep without interruption. I almost chucked his C-PAP prescription in the hallway trash barrel when I remembered the look on my ma's face as she handed me the Dear Abby article. I also remembered the fact that my wife deserved better than to become a widow because her husband ate himself to death. Heck, if I was going out, I wanted to go in a blaze of glory, not by way of some obscure sleep disorder. Later, I learned that it wasn't all that obscure. In fact, a huge amount of our population, regardless of their weight, is affected by Sleep Apnea.

The day after meeting with my doctor I sat with my arms folded at Lincare, Inc. in Woburn, MA, while a nice guy named Chris casually described how easy the C-PAP machine was to use. My mood was a mixture of disgust (that medical science hadn't invented a better treatment for Sleep Apnea) and sarcasm (that anyone actually thought someone as young as I was going to sleep with a Darth Vader setup strapped to his face).

"You mean to tell me that people are actually wearing these to bed every night?" I asked Chris.

"You bet," he said. "We're distributing a huge amount of these machines every week." I remember thinking to myself, *Save your sales spiel, mine's going right to the back of the closet.* I was 31 years old. This was for someone at the "Last Stop Care Facility" up the street.

"I'm a young guy with a weight problem. Am I really expected to get into bed every night with my wife while I'm wearing one of these?" I asked.

"Plenty of people do. It's a matter of life or death," Chris responded.

"Hey, Honey, wanna play that kinky Star Wars game again tonight?" I mockingly joked with Chris.

As Chris fit my face for the right headgear, my eyes focused on a poster on the wall in his office. It was an advertisement by one of the C-PAP manufacturers. In the picture, the four US presidents on Mount Rushmore were wearing C-PAP masks. Cute advertisement, but it began to haunt me. *Sleeping with a C-PAP is now supposed to be viewed as a pure slice of Americana. Like Mom and apple pie? Was this really what our forefathers had in mind?* It seemed to me that like countless other medical problems, we were treating the symptoms with a band-aid instead of dealing with the causes of the problem in the first place.

Chris continued his C-PAP tour.

"Okay, so this hose connects to this plastic joint, which is then connected to the face mask," he explained. "The Velcro is then spooled through and connected to the sides of the mask. Then pull it over your head like so. Be sure to wash your face every night before putting it on. Then once a week dismantle the mask piece-by-piece and wash it in warm water in the sink. The headgear can go in the washing machine." At this point I was all about selective ADD, the version of attention deficit disorder where you simply tune out what you could care less about.

When I rejoined the conversation, Chris was still telling me more about C-PAPs than I ever wanted to know. The machine itself was small, and it was attached to a long medical-style hose that connected to a clear plastic face mask that covered the nose and mouth.

All things considered, the gizmo reeked of life support and I would have none of it. I refused to give my family and friends the satisfaction of having to sleep with a breathing machine because of the weight problem they'd lectured me about for an entire lifetime.

As I left the Lincare Facility, I decided that the machine would never live to see even the back of my closet, so I stashed it in the back of my car trunk for the next 2½ years.

During that time period the disease intensified and all of my family inquired about the C-PAP machine. "Don't you have to sleep with an oxygen machine or something?" asked my brother.

"Isn't it dangerous for you not to be using that machine?" asked Rainbow more than a few times.

"Nope, I'm fine without it," I'd answer with slightly annoyed pride.

I forged on with my life, the whole time with this machine in my car next to my portable cooler. One time, following a lunch meeting, an actress client of mine noticed the C-PAP hose in my trunk and gave me a strange look. "What's that thing? she asked with a disturbed curiosity in her voice.

"Trust me, you don't want to know," I responded as I jammed it further back into my car's trunk. Later it occurred to me that the poor girl probably thought I was into something kinky like asphyxiation or something. But in truth, I was happier with her thinking that.

◆　　　◆　　　◆

Time moves on, whether you are conscious or sleeping. As the C-PAP collected dust and gas fumes in my truck, my mild case of Obstructive Sleep Apnea worsened. By 1998 it had become severe. My days at that time consisted of waking up exhausted around 8:00 a.m., dragging myself to the office, then napping by late morning and napping again in the early and mid afternoon. I began to lose track of significant work details, and even more disastrously, began falling asleep during phone calls and in the middle of client meetings. Charming, huh? One time during the taping of an interview with an expert on Y2K, I fell asleep and began snoring loudly. The director and cameraman did their best to cover up the fact that I was asleep in the back of the room. *"Okay, let's try the intro one more time,"* they shouted in an obvious and loud tone of voice. *"All right, I like that last take. What do you think, Mr. Director?"* they yelled as they jabbed me in the side.

Another time, in a pre-production meeting, a client asked me if I recalled anything she'd said in the last 15 minutes. I responded that I did, but when she quizzed me about specifics it was apparent that I was out if it. "C'mon Gary," she said in a panic. "Our project deadline is in one week!" I could care less. All I wanted was to throw her off my couch so I could sleep. Things were left undone at work and my declining health was hardly lost on my clients. It wasn't lost on them because I was falling asleep with them everyday while on the phone. You could hear the concern in their voices. *Okay, it sounds like you're fading again…can you hear me now…okay, how about now?*

Nor was it lost on them that I was losing focus when it came to their careers. Occasionally, acts I was representing would drop by my office and suggest we take a walk. "Have you ever heard of an organization called [*insert weight loss group/12-step program here*]?" I could sense they were generally concerned for my health and I'd graciously accept their advice, then head back to bed, which was all I really ever cared about.

I did my best to function with the disorder, but my conscious mind was fading in and out, blurring the days into nights. And that wasn't the worst of it. Statistically the majority of Sleep Apnea cases were being diagnosed following auto accidents (people falling asleep behind the wheel) and my driving was beginning to resemble Mr. Magoo's. Friends and co-workers began to grow wary of riding with me. The scenario was always the same: we'd get in the car and begin talking about issues that were at hand. Eventually they would notice that I was not responding and I'd begin weaving in and out of the lanes. Whatever energy I had was used to keep my eyes open. I could barely hold onto the wheel. People were scared, and who could blame them? Near-accidents and close calls were becoming daily occurrences. Rather than use the machine in my trunk, I simply accepted these potentially fatal accidents as a fact of life. I also accepted the roadside naps that became daily rituals. Whether I was alone or with Julie, I was always pulling over. Burger King. Roy Rogers. The weigh station. You name it, I slept there. There I'd be in recline position, snorting and wheezing like a champ. It was an awful way to live, and I believe to this day that an angel somewhere was looking out for me through all of it. By all rights, Sleep Apnea should have been written on my death certificate. In fact, by the summer of that year I became resigned to the fact that I was slowly dying. I can remember pushing my nieces, Alexandra,

Mackenzie, Isabella and Brette, as well as my nephew Chris on the swings at my sister's house and thinking how much I would regret not being around to see them become adults. I was at peace with it. By this point I only wanted to lie down and sleep. The sleeping became a part of my personality; people expected it and joked about it. One Christmas Eve I fell asleep at my friend Vinnie's house in Stow, MA. While I slept, he videotaped me. Eventually I awoke and he played the tape back for me. It was one of the most disturbing things I ever watched. That snoring was loud, man! And I was struggling to breathe correctly throughout the videotape. I found the tape so hard to watch that I erased it immediately. I just didn't want it to exist. If I could find the ones from my sleep study, I'd have erased those as well. Keeping my disorder under wraps was important to me. As a result, my friends and relatives never quite realized the severity of the disorder. Instead, they looked for the humor in my narcoleptic ways. Many times I'd fall asleep on their couches. When I awoke, I'd be buried underneath a heap of stuffed animals. Eventually they'd show me Polaroid photos they'd taken of me sleeping on the couch, surrounded by the toys. At the time the photos were funny, but when I looked closely at the images, the scenes weren't so funny. I stuffed the photos away in my luggage and didn't find them until that fateful night in July of 1998 when I and my car nearly went crashing into the Atlantic Ocean near Falmouth. I don't actually know what made me reach underneath my seat that night, but the next thing I knew, I was holding those Kodak memories in my hand. The salt in the ocean water—which I had just narrowly avoided—had nothing on the salt in my tears that night. I tried to reflect on my life and how to regain control of it, but as I stared out at the tiny lights of Martha's Vineyard, I began to fade again, and this time it was for the night.

◆   ◆   ◆

I showed up at the boat dock the next morning just as Julie, my cousin Michele and my Uncle Dave's family were all loading their bags and coolers onto the boat. I kissed Julie, and I jumped right in to help, apologizing for not arriving the night before as promised. "I worked late and left this morning," I explained, deciding to spare them the story of my near-death experience. We had planned a day of swimming and boating over in Vineyard Haven, about a half hour ride from Falmouth. Shortly after untying the boat and leaving the dock I headed down below to sleep in the cabin for the entire 30-minute ride to Martha's Vineyard. Once the boat was anchored in the flats (I wasn't awake to assist with any of that) I jumped into a small life raft, which was tied off the back of the boat with 30 feet of slack. Once again, I immediately passed out and baked in the sun for the remainder of day. As I slept, my family engaged in their usual water ball games and diving competitions while loud music blared from the boat's eight speakers. When I finally came to, it was nearly 4:00 p.m. and time to go back to the mainland. I'd missed another entire day's worth of fun with my family, and it couldn't have gone unnoticed by them. I helped pull the anchor up, made a quick cold-cut sandwich, and returned to my solitary sleep in the cabin below until we arrived back at the dock in Falmouth. After a shower at the Cape house, Uncle Dave and I cooked dinner on the grill for everyone (my one contribution to the family get-togethers) and then I fell asleep on the couch for more of those creative Polaroids. Eventually, bedtime came for everyone, and I retired along with them at around 10:00 p.m. However, I was completely unaware that the most horrific wake-up call of my life was just around the corner.

POST-TRAUMATIC
STRETCH DISORDER:
Death of a Rainbow

"Life's not only for the living, it's what you leave behind."

—*Brad Delp*

I woke up on a late August afternoon, face down on the couch in my office. The phone on my desk was ringing, but in my Sleep Apnea coma I could not find the energy to get up. The phone continued to ring, and I wondered when someone was going to answer it. It finally occurred to me that I had let my assistant go home early that day, so no one was covering my phones. I rolled onto the floor, balanced myself on my knees and knocked half of the stuff off my desk while reaching for the phone. "Gary Marino," I answered energetically. By this time I was a pro at sounding alert, even though I had just woken up.

"Gary, it's Rich. I've got some bad news about Ma that is going to knock the wind out of your sails," said my brother. I could tell the gravity of the situation by the tone of his voice. "Dad noticed Ma was having trouble walking and talking this morning. He brought her to the hospital for some tests. They've found a large tumor in her brain and are prepping her for immediate surgery."

I sat back against the wall, holding the phone in silent shock. After two and a half years battling Obstructive Sleep Apnea, I was suddenly more awake than I'd been in a long time. I could not respond to the news, but in many ways it all made sense. My folks had been living in London, England, as part of my dad's new job, handling marketing for his company's European operation. In June of 1998 he and my mom had returned home to Boston permanently to retire. Strangely, Rainbow's trademark smile and warm personality had been replaced by confusion, nervousness and panic attacks. My siblings and I were deeply concerned, but assumed that the change of lifestyles from the U.K. to the U.S.A. were to blame. As the summer rolled on, it became apparent that my mom's condition was getting worse, not better. Rainbow had gone from an incredibly young, hip and at ease 59-year-old to acting like a woman in her 90s. The news of the brain tumor was numbing, but again I had to admit it all made sense. I immediately made my way to Massachusetts General Hospital, where my mom, looking brave and beautiful, lay in bed, ready to face the surgery. Like most families dealing with cancer for the first time, we were aware of the seriousness of my mother's situation, but certain that the surgery would successfully remove the tumor. Perhaps chemotherapy would be needed in conjunction with the surgery, but we believed that eventually Rainbow would return home with a new and healthy lease on life. How naïve we were.

As I began overdosing on comfort foods to calm my nerves, my wife Julie wisely began hitting the Internet to research the type of tumor my ma had. She printed many documents with which I was able to educate myself so I could read between the lines of what the doctors and my dad were saying. Perhaps they were trying to protect us, but based on the disturbing information Julie found for me, my mother's situation was grave. Rainbow had a grade-four malignant glioblastoma lodged in her brain behind her right temple. Most folks with my mother's type of tumor had 6 to 18 months to live. Surgery and chemotherapy were time-buying measures at best.

I closed my eyes and invited denial into my mind. All I hoped was that my sweet, selfless and innocent mother would live to enjoy her richly-deserved retirement and watch her wonderful grandchildren grow up. I refused to believe that Ma would never meet my own children and be a part of their lives, the same way her mother had been a part of mine. I also refused to believe that my mother would not be around to see me conquer my life-long weight problem—a promise I had made to her for the better part of 15 years. As much as it hurt, I showed the documents to my brother and sisters. Their reaction mirrored mine, which was, *I don't want to read this.*

Rainbow bravely and courageously faced her surgery and chemotherapy sessions, determined to buy more time. Throughout everything that fall, family and friends flocked to my mother's side, driving her to hospital visits and providing whatever else she needed. I spent quality time with Rainbow during those months, cutting way back on my work schedule so I could take her for long walks or support her during trips to Mass General. Of course by this point my Sleep Apnea kept me in a permanent state of exhaustion, and many times, while taking care of my mother, I actually fell asleep in her presence. I often woke up to find myself covered with a blanket, and her sleeping uncovered on a nearby couch. A mother until the end.

As October and November of 1998 dragged on, my mom seemed to slowly slip away with each day that passed—a little less physical ability and a little more confusion mentally. Even with this, our family refused to believe that we were actually losing Rainbow. There were, of course, miracle cases in all those statistics Julie was finding, and we were determined that Ma was going to be one of them. I continued to eat self-destructively and ignore my own declining health, but not my mother's.

On Christmas Day, 1998, I volunteered to stay home alone with Ma while the family held a holiday get-together at my sister Donna's home in Windham, New Hampshire. On that day Rainbow seemed quiet, reserved and unresponsive. On a trip to take her to the bathroom, she collapsed in my arms. I frantically phoned 911 as my mother lay on the floor of the bathroom, unconscious. It was one of those awful, surreal moments that you never quite get over. The ambulance arrived and I rode with Ma back to Mass General. When we arrived, most of the family was waiting there, stunned and silent. We all stayed with my ma, who seemed low-key and confused until the doctors arrived at 3:00 a.m. Clearly the tumor had grown back, but the extent of the damage would not be known until additional tests were performed. Between what had just happened and my own sleep deprivation, I was ready to drop. I decided to head back to my apartment to get some sleep, leaving the rest of the family with Ma. The next morning, around 10:00 a.m., a knock at the door woke me from yet another coma-like sleep. I dragged myself over to the door and looked in the peephole to see who it was. The sad, tired faces of my brother and two sisters said it all. A quiet heaviness filled the air as they followed me into the dining room to sit down. I looked around. Clothes were piled everywhere. Boxes were stacked against the walls. CD cases, videotapes, paperwork and junk littered the room. Before I could become too embarrassed, my siblings announced the news. "The doctors saw Ma this morning, looked at her CT scan results and told us that there is nothing more they can do. Her health will only go downhill from here. They estimate 3 weeks to 2 months to live." Once again I found myself speechless. I reached around and grabbed a photo of Rainbow with the four of us in the early 1970s. There was Ma in all her glory, proudly posing with her kids. She seemed to smile back at me at that moment. The room was stone-cold quiet. I stood up, walked around the table, grabbed my brother and sisters and we cried and hugged for what seemed an eternity. Suddenly, my thoughts turned towards the hospital.

"Who is with her now?" I asked.

"Dad was when we left. He wanted to be alone with her, then he was going to go home and take a shower," my sister answered.

"I'll head up in case she's alone," I said as I walked them to the door.

We hugged one more time before they left. Being with my brother and sisters made me feel complete, almost as if Ma was okay, but when they left I broke down in a way in which I never have before. I guess you could say it was my first experience with total despondency. I cried loudly, hysterically, and uncontrollably at the true realization that my mother was going to die and there was nothing I could do about it. I cursed God in one breath and then laughed at some of the funny times Ma and I shared together in the next. I rolled on the floor, wailing in despair, and threw furniture against the walls in protest. I got on my knees and begged God through my tears to somehow miraculously save her. I offered my own life if He could just spare hers, and then laughed like a crazy person for thinking I could actually cut a deal. This wasn't the movies. This was the cold, raw reality of life. She was going to go and there was nothing I could do about it. To this day I will never forget that feeling of total helplessness and solitude.

◆   ◆   ◆

We moved Ma a week later to a Transitional Care Unit at Lawrence Memorial Hospital in Medford. A very fitting place, actually, not far from the schools where she volunteered and the parks where she took us in our formative years. Although there were times when my mom was lucid, for the most part she began sleeping more and eating and responding less. Although the family braced for the reality we knew would come, we never gave up hope that some miracle might occur and the tumor which had now wrapped itself around my ma's brain stem might suddenly begin shrinking on it's own. As January dragged into February, countless friends and family, touched by my ma's legacy of unselfish giving and unconditional love, descended upon her hospital room. The doctors at the Transitional Care Unit were amazed that my mother was still hanging on at this point, but they assured us that she was near the end. The family broke up into shifts so Rainbow would never be alone. In the early morning hours of February 6, 1999, I awoke in an adjacent recreational room across the hall from my mother's. Something told me that the hour had come—one of those strange feelings where you just know. As I sat up in the uncomfortable chair, I stopped to watch my sister Donna (she was doing the overnight shift with me) sleeping quite comfortably in the chair across from me. Donna looked adorable, all folded up in a deep sleep, looking like one of her young daughters. Watching her, I felt grateful that she had given our mother four wonderful grandchildren. I hoped she was proud of the kind of daughter she was.

"Donna, wake up," I whispered. "I think we should check on Ma."

As Donna and I walked across the hall, a nurse ran out of my mother's room. "She's going now," she said. We rushed to her bedside...

Ma passed.

Donna held her hand as I closed her beautiful hazel green eyes. "Sleep with angels," my sister told our mother as she slipped away. Just five months after being diagnosed with brain cancer, Rainbow was gone forever. For the last time, the family gathered in my mother's hospital room. There we stayed with her body for two more hours, both crying and laughing about the times we had together. In its own way, it was beautiful.

At 5:00 a.m. we said our final good-byes to Rainbow and wearily headed back to my folks' home by the lake in West Medford. Exhausted and knowing I'd need my energy, I bid goodnight to everyone and headed toward the stairs that led up to my old bedroom. As I walked past the front door, something caught my eye. February 6, 1999 was a typical cold, cloudy, overcast winter day in New England, but for some reason a gorgeous pink and orange sun stretched across the morning sky. It was so blinding that I called my family out onto the front lawn to observe what was happening. We had never seen anything like it in our region at that time of the year. "There's Ma," I said, as we all marveled at the colors bursting from the sky. Heaven had its prized angel back. A reunion was taking place, the likes of which we could only imagine. She had gone home. All we could do was stand there and smile.

◆   ◆   ◆

Ma's wake and funeral were a testament to her impact on people's lives. The lines outside of the funeral home went out of the building, onto the street, down a side street and around the block. Uncle Dave joked that Rainbow had "sold out" the funeral home. Two police motorcycles escorted the hearses. At St. Joseph's Church, where my mother had attended Mass for years, Catholic priests and Jesuits came together and customized a one-of-a-kind funeral for her. At her burial at Oak Grove Cemetery, Dad, myself and my three siblings symbolically released five white balloons into the air. The huge crowd around the gravesite began to clap their hands loudly and applaud my mother's life. Let's face it, when people are applauding you at your burial, you know you've done something right.

Life is never the same after you lose your mom, but as hard as it was, the day came when everybody needed to go back to their lives and attempt to move on. I returned to my office the following week to see how my company had fared during my 4-5 week hiatus. Business had gone remarkably well. Despite everything and in spite of myself, Harmon-Marino seemed poised to have its best year ever. The growing list of independent contractors now working for us had doubled in a two-year period. My health, however, was beginning to bottom out. The Sleep Apnea by this point had me where it wanted me, and my life truly had become days of nights.

As 1999 moved on, Post-Traumatic Stretch Disorder—or what some call emotional eating—went into overdrive. It seemed to be the case for most of the family. Maybe it was the shock of losing Ma 20 years before her time. Or perhaps it was the sight of my father, brave as he was, alone and wearing his dark "*Aristotle Onassis, I'm in mourning 24/7*" glasses. We were truly a family adrift in depression. For years I'd promised Rainbow that I would lose the weight and get healthy. It had been her dream to see me fit and happy. Now I was faced with the reality that she'd never see it. As life-changing as her death was, I still could not find the motivation I needed to turn the situation around. I'd always joked with my wife that when the day came my mother passed, my taste buds would magically go numb. But as March turned into April, it was apparent that I was eating even more, not less. I had no idea what I weighed by that time, but judging from the way I felt, I was sure I'd manage to gain even more weight. At work we ordered Chinese food, pizza, and subs the size of your forearm. Julie and I at that point were living in a run-down temporary apartment I had dubbed "Hell's Kitchen," where we ate (you guessed it) take out Chinese food, pizza and subs. No meals were ever cooked there due to the lack of a good, clean and inviting kitchen, so as a result 99% of the meals I was eating were at restaurants or at work. In the mirror and in photos I looked like a guy exhausted and blatantly uncomfortable in his own body, a bloated caricature of a human so very lost. The last time I had been on an actual scale was during an office pool I had going with some of the guys in my office to lose weight. That was two years earlier and after weighing in at 376 pounds, I'd abruptly quit the competition, deciding I needed more than a cutesy "let's see who can lose the most weight" type of contest to turn things around. That stuff had all become old to me. I was well aware that my situation would require drastic measures. All I ever seemed to want to do was sleep. How I managed to keep my business afloat I have no idea to this day. Julie and I decided that a year in "Hell's Kitchen" was enough, so in June we purchased a clean, spacious and relatively new condominium in West Woburn, about a mile from my office in Burlington. The quiet complex was surrounded by woods. I hired a moving company to move our stuff, knowing that I was incapable of performing anything too physical. As the sleep disorder completely zapped my energy, the circles around my eyes darkened. I wore loose, style-deprived clothes that looked sloppy and uncomfortable. Family and friends stood by, helplessly watching my health decline.

One morning, not long after we moved into the condo, Julie woke me from a sound sleep. "Did you leave the stereo on when you went to bed last night?" she asked.

I could barely open my eyes. "Not that I remember," I answered. Of course at that point, Julie and I were both aware that anything was possible in my confused, sleep-deprived state of mind.

"That's weird, because it's playing in the living room and the volume is pretty loud," she said. Julie and I dismissed the incident as a Sleep Apnea thing. The next morning, however, as she got dressed for work, my wife noticed the stereo was on once again. "Can you believe it? It's playing again!" she said alarmingly. We theorized that it had to be a power surge in the building. Around 3:00 a.m. on the third night, I awoke from my loud snoring and snorting routine and headed for the bathroom. On my way back I stared down the long dark hallway leading to the living room. It was eerie and quiet. I'd been reading books about spirituality in the months since Ma's death, and most seemed to suggest that the deceased could send signs by turning on electrical devices such as TVs and stereos. "What are you going to do tonight, Ma, play me a CD?" I said as I looked to my right into the blackness of the hallway. I crawled into bed and as my head hit the pillow, an old Dusty Springfield song came on in the living room. I sat straight up, shaken. "Jules, wake up! Do you hear that? The stereo's on again!" I yelled. Now I've always believed in the paranormal, but this was beginning to even wig me out. Julie and I nervously made our way in the darkness to the living room. There on the CD player was my wife's Dusty Springfield disc playing loudly. Now I was freaked out for two reasons. First that my wife actually owned a Dusty Springfield CD, and second that the stereo turned itself on when I dared it to do so. I loved our new condo, but the stereo poltergeist was really beginning to wreak havoc on my brain. You can believe in the afterlife all you want, folks, but trust me, when you get real signs it still startles you. By the fourth night, I began playing with the stereo a bit. I pulled all the CDs and cassettes out of it and took it out of stereo mode. That night the stereo was playing again. The following night I decided to eliminate the possibility of a power surge by turning the volume completely down and muting it as well. At 3:00 a.m. the stereo woke me up. This time I collapsed into a chair in front of it and slapped the power off. "What do you think is doing this?" I asked my wife in a disturbed tone.

"Maybe it's your mother, sending you a sign about your Sleep Apnea," Julie theorized.

"That's cute, Hon. Are you suggesting that I'm actually stressing my mother out from beyond the grave?" I responded.

"Maybe," Julie answered.

For the next three weeks the stereo continued it's 3:00 a.m. routine. By the end I was begging my mother, if in fact it was her, to let me sleep an entire night through. I was sleep deprived as it was. In July I entered the Bedford Sleep Center for yet another sleep study. This time the results seemed to show that the disease had in fact reached a life-threatening point.

"I would be very concerned if you were a relative of mine," said the sleep specialist as she scrutinized my results. "Your heart rate drops way off and then shoots back up dozens of times a night." In the morning she asked whether or not I'd been using a C-PAP. I responded that I might be open to it at this point. Just to give me a feel for it, she slapped a C-PAP mask on my face and turned the sample unit on. I fell asleep right there in her office. It was so peaceful. Later that day I dug the unit out of my trunk from two and a half years earlier and put it on that very night. I slept straight through the night. No stereo. The next night I did the same thing. No stereo. By the third night I felt like a new man. I felt giddy, energetic and full of new life. I laughed for the first time in months. I accepted that I would use the C-PAP until the day came when I lost the weight. I vowed that I would not sleep with the machine forever. I would use it as inspiration to get healthy.

"And what about that stereo poltergeist problem?" you ask. Well, it never happened again after the night I entered the sleep clinic. As the summer of 1999 dragged on, I willed it, dared it and taunted it, but it never turned itself on again. Believe what you want to believe. Everyone is entitled to his or her own opinion. But for me, my mother saved my life that summer. A mother till the end and even now, years after her death. Energy does not die. And love, particularly a mother's love, is truly forever. By December, a fresh snow had fallen around her rose quartz gravestone. In the snow I wrote the words "Rainbow lives." For me, she always will.

10,000 CHEESEBURGERS IN PARADISE

"So do you super-size at the drive thru or just let them go with the assumption?"

—Conan O'Brien

In December of 1999, Julie and I flew to Hawaii to celebrate the coming of the new millennium and to take in some long overdue rest. At this point I'd been putting in16-hour days, trying to get everything done business-wise before we left. We rented a beach house in Wailea with Uncle David, his wife Karen, their daughter Devyn, and my cousin Michele.

Michele was Rainbow's niece, and the two of us had formed a special relationship following the recent deaths of both of our mothers, due to cancer. Michele is the youngest of six, about four years younger than I. While our age difference isn't dramatic, I'd never gotten to know her especially well when we were growing up. When we finally bonded in the summers of 1998 and 1999, we were amazed at how similar we were in terms of the kinds of relationships we seek out in others, the humorous outlooks we have on the world, and—you guessed it—food! Somehow I managed to find a female complement in Michele and she soon became the closest thing I'd ever had to a twin, right down to completing each other's thoughts and sentences, a ritual that would really wig our spouses out. Michele and I were one, all right, and it didn't stop with our idiosyncrasies. My cousin had the food addict thing going as well, but to her credit, she'd managed to keep it somewhat in check. Michele might have had a few pounds to lose, but physically she was a blonde, blue-eyed head turner. For me it was like meeting Rainbow and Ida as thirty-year-olds. Michele possessed the best of both of their personalities. The good news was that Michele was joining us in Maui. The bad news? The flight was fourteen hours total.

Two hours from Boston to Chicago, then a five-hour connecting flight to San Francisco, followed by a two-hour layover before boarding yet another flight to the island of Maui, which was another seven hours away. Never in a million years did I think that all this flying would be easy for a *man of girth* like myself. At this point in my life I'd become convinced that Ethiopians had designed airplane seats. In preparation, I packed my carry-on with as many over-the-counter pain killers as I could in order to numb the pain I knew I'd be experiencing from wedging myself into the seat. It was a beautiful, clear, crisp December morning. My production company had just finished a banner year and I was heading for Hawaii for nearly three weeks. I remember telling myself that "flying in a tightly packed airplane is not enough to spoil the mood I'm in."

We boarded a 747 for the first leg of the trip and the scene was the same as it always had been. I made my way down the center aisle with my carry-on bag and cup of coffee, trying to concentrate on counting the rows of seats instead of the anxious looks I got from each of the seated passengers as I passed by. Some literally looked like they'd seen a ghost. I thought to myself, *Relax folks, I've got my wife with me. She'll work as a buffer between us. How bad can it be?* As we made our way down into the bowels of the plane, the looks went from "heightened alert" to downright scared. *No need to worry, my troubled countrymen, I'm deceptively compact for a man of girth.*

By the time we found our seats in the back of the plane, it dawned on me that political correctness—America's theme of sensitivity throughout the 1990s—had been lost on the entire "Fat" thing. Not that I was asking to be seen as "aerobically challenged," but how about hiding your uneasiness concerning the idea of sharing a seat? If the country wasn't more compassionate at this point, I doubted that it ever would be. Julie took the center seat, as always, so I could have the aisle seat. Oh yeah, the aisle seat. It's like hitting the lottery for the big guys out there!

Once I was in my Ally McBeal designer seat, I knew the routine. Take a deep breath and jam the seat belt closed, or flag down the flight attendant and ask for an extension belt. Great system, folks. Why don't we just slap a bumper sticker over my lap that says "Wide Load"? From there the flight went smoothly, except for the occasional moments when I would fall asleep and wake up abruptly with loud Sleep Apnea snorts that would shock the entire cabin. Ah, the life of an overweight traveler! Next up, lunch time. Something I was supposed to be skilled at, but when I unlocked the dinner tray on the seat in front of me, it sat diagonally at a 45-degree angle on my stomach. I quickly snapped it back into place.

By the three-hour mark, I was looking for any distraction I could find. My legs had gone numb, and I seemed to be getting bumped in the shoulder by every single—and I'm not exaggerating here—every single person heading to the bathroom in the back of the plane. Talk about Chinese torture! Finally, a viable distraction presented itself. The flight attendant announced that the in-flight movie, a Disney film for kids, would be starting in 5 minutes. *Great. I don't even care what it is. Just give me something to get my mind off the pain,* I thought. *I'll watch a "Murder She Wrote" marathon, a double episode of Matlock. I don't care.*

"You'll find your headsets conveniently located in the seat pocket in front of you," the flight attendant announced. I found my headset easily enough and slipped it on just as the movie started. Just one problem. I could not find the jack where the headset plugged in. I looked up, down, left, right, you name it. I literally scoured the seat to find the port. It was now a full ten minutes into the movie and everybody was in the recline position watching this stupid film. Exasperated, I flagged down a flight attendant.

"Excuse me, miss? Can you please tell me where exactly this headset plugs in?" I asked.

She smiled and very professionally answered, "Why of course, sir. The audio input is located on the underside and toward the back of your armrest."

Now I looked at her even more confused. "Armrest?" I asked. "Where the hell is there an armrest here? Do you see an armrest?" Eventually I realized the armrest was completely covered by my girth, which in turn was covered by my loud and over-sized Hawaiian shirt. *Who the hell wants to watch some stupid kid's movie anyway?* I asked myself. *After all, there's only, what, ten, eleven hours of flying left?*

The Island of Maui was a paradise like nothing I'd ever experienced before. Lush green valleys, gorgeous beaches with white sand and aquamarine water, mountains that disappeared into the sky and weather so perfect you'd swear you were on a climate-controlled movie set somewhere. We snorkeled in Molokai, beached it all day in Kihei and watched the sunrise beneath the clouds over the mountain of Haleakala. I was truly on a mission to experience it all in Hawaii, and that mission wasn't limited to sight-seeing activities. About a week into the trip, I bumped into a place downtown which featured an "All You Can Eat" cheeseburger buffet. The restaurant name was pretty bland, so I nick-named it "10,000 Cheeseburgers in Paradise." What's in a name, anyway, when we're talking about a restaurant dedicated to the art of the cheeseburger? The place featured five different types of seasoned ground sirloin, fifteen different types of cheese, and seven choices of fresh rolls, ranging from onion bulkie, poppyseed to Portuguese sweet roll. The "dressings" bar ran the length of the place and offered an abundance of pickles, lettuce, assorted peppers, Vidalia onion wedges, red and green relishes, green and red ketchup, mayonnaise, yellow mustard, honey mustard, and tangy Dijon mustard. All pure rapture to a cheeseburger lover.

I dragged Julie to the cheeseburger buffet every other day, and with each stop the burgers got bigger, tastier and, well, more creative. Monday I had the 6-ounce Teriyaki burger with salsa, followed up by a classic 8-ounce American cheeseburger with BBQ sauce, bacon, and sautéed onions, all on a sweet roll. Even a traditional vegetarian would break ranks for one of my 10 oz. Swiss cheeseburgers with ketchup, relish, mustard, mayo, pickles, lettuce, and tomatoes. And dare I mention, all of this on a sesame seed bun? Maui was heaven, all right, and occasionally I made excuses to head into town to experience yet another pass at paradise by the buffet lights. "I'm heading downtown to pick up a few things, does anyone need anything?" I'd ask. Talk about a scene from "Honey, I Blew Up The Speedo."

Eventually, I turned my thoughts away from cheeseburgers and toward the upcoming new millennium. On December 31 our entire gang celebrated with a New Year's Eve luau at the Grand Wailea Resort, one of the top three resorts in the world at the time. As the final moments of the 20th century wound down, a sudden feeling of melancholy came over me. A brand new century was starting, and as usual, I couldn't make a fresh start of anything because of the same problem that had been dogging me my entire life. I was still the fat kid at war with himself, trying to live a good life and do good things, but even at 33, I felt angry and trapped every step of the way. Even in Maui, with all of its heavenly beauty, I was in hell. On the beach I felt embarrassed and sedentary. When we snorkeled, I felt bloated and uncomfortable in the equipment. In the outrageous beachfront restaurants I struggled to be comfortable in chairs that were too small and gorged myself into a food funk.

Before I left for Maui, I had confessed to a close buddy of mine how much I was dreading the 14-hour flight to Hawaii. He seized the moment to have a sincere conversation with me. "You could win the lottery tomorrow, Gary, fly to any island paradise you wanted, and you'd still be in Hell, looking and feeling the way you do," he said frankly. Harsh words, but in Maui his statement became eerily true. I was physically standing in Heaven but mentally drowning in Hell. I'd spent nearly $10,000 on this trip but hadn't really enjoyed a penny's worth. It was hard not to feel alienated—from everything.

Then one night, toward the end of our vacation, my uncle and I were sitting on the deck of our rented house in Maui, sipping iced tea and watching the breathtaking sunset. We'd just wrapped up dinner and the girls had gone downtown to shop. As we watched the sun disappear into the ocean, we began talking about, what else, our weight. At the time my uncle was in his 50s and finally beginning to get control of his own life-long weight problem. He'd recently been diagnosed with Type two diabetes and was warning me to control my weight problem before the disease came knocking down my door as well. I was an old pro at these conversations by now. As I described my current defeatist attitude towards losing weight, he asked me a question that caught me off guard.

"At this point in your life," he asked me, "what are the pros to your being overweight, and what are the cons you live with everyday as a result?"

I had to think hard about that one. *Maybe*, I thought, *I should think about it over dessert.* No. I could see that he was genuinely interested in my answer and not simply making "fat talk" for the heck of it. I'd never really thought about it in those terms, you know? Then, for the first time in my life, I gave someone a completely honest answer. I said, "Here's the only pro of being overweight. I can eat anything, anywhere, anytime I want. I never have to deny myself, I never have to think about it, and I don't count calories or watch fat grams. I can have as much as I want of anything. No one is policing me or stopping me. Life is a paradise under the buffet lights."

"Okay," he said, nodding his head, as if my answer actually had some merit. "What are the cons?" I carefully gathered my thoughts and answered. "The cons are everything else, Uncle. As a result of being overweight I'm screwed in everything I try to do in life, everything from A to Z." My uncle didn't react. He left me to die with my own material, as some of my comedian clients might say.

"I'm gonna go put on some Kona coffee." he said. I sat there in the dark, staring at the faded sunset. I don't remember how long I stayed out there thinking about what I had just admitted to myself. The one perk, the one pathetic thing I got for my present condition was the ability to gorge myself everyday. Big deal. As a result, in everything else I attempted to do in life—whether it be sports, relationships, work, or simple things like walking down the beach or buying jeans off the rack—I was royally screwed. I thought about everything I'd been through and the awful way my weight had affected my life. I thought of the awful solitude I encountered as a result of never being able to fix myself and the verbal and mental daggers I had been dealing with my whole life. *Maybe it's time to leave this problem behind in the twentieth century,* I thought. *I'm 33, for God's sake. Half my life is over.*

On the return flight from San Francisco to Boston, something unique happened. The plane was only half-filled. To most thin people it was not a big deal, but to people my size it was like Christmas. Leg room, head room, a row to one's self, it might as well be a flying Jacuzzi to us.

I separated from my wife (she'd caught enough of my act in Hawaii) and found a row to myself about halfway back into the plane. Suddenly a young kid's head popped up next to me and said, "I'm Mario, what's your name?"

"Gary," I said as I gave him the traditional "be a good kid and shut up now" pat on the head.

Initially I was not happy about having someone sitting next to me, but something about this kid was engaging. The kid was a chubby little 11-year-old chatterbox. He wore shorts and a loose "It's better in Hawaii" tee shirt over the rolls of baby fat that still hung around his stomach. He was amusingly upbeat and explained to me that he, too, was from Boston and that his family was sitting in the seats behind us. I turned to look behind me to say "hi" to Mario's family. They shook my hand and rolled their eyes, almost as if to say "we know, we know, the kid talks nonstop, that's why we're all sitting back here.'

Mario wasted no time in telling me about his trip to Hawaii. "Swam with the turtles in Kapalua, saw the sharks up close at the Maui Ocean Center and counted twenty-two whales off the coast of Kanapali. Twenty-two! Did you see any?" he asked.

"Lots, you bet," I said and nodded. The kid was adorable and full of wonderment, but something about him made my heart sink. He was thoroughly overweight, yet youthfully optimistic, full of personality and fascinated with his world in a way that only a kid can be. Suddenly I wasn't bummed out about having to share my row with someone. My neck was craned for hours and Mario never seemed to stop chit-chatting.

"The family didn't want to do a helicopter ride," he went on, "but I wanted to see where they filmed Star Wars. Did ya see the volcano?" I pretty much tuned the kid out half way through the flight back to Boston, yet I couldn't take my eyes off of him. I knew exactly what this kid would go through as he grew up. The challenge just to find clothes that fit, the insults he'd endure, and the way people would treat him like a second-class citizen. The way his guy friends would take advantage of every cheap shot they could and the way the women would dismiss him as a crude joke. The kid wouldn't have a chance. A part of me wished I could go home with him, make a friend of him, and help him figure out what I was only just beginning to figure out for myself, which is that a quality life was impossible for a fat person in the year 2000. *It would be the equivalent of saving the kid from a "waisted youth,"* I thought. Halfway through the flight, the kid was still going strong. "My dad wouldn't let me too close to the whales," he continued, "but I wanted to take a picture of one. Did you ever see the movie 'Free Willy'?" I wanted to *Free Gary* by that point, but I couldn't stop thinking about what this chubby, East Boston kid's life would be like in the years to come. Would he keep his upbeat personality and fascination with life? Or would he slowly grow jaded and angry, frustrated at his inability to develop his life properly? I knew those frustrations all too well, and watching and listening to him made me feel like I was meeting myself as an 11-year-old. While the rest of the airplane may have considered Mario just an overweight Italian boy, what I saw was a young person who would have three times the normal risk for type two diabetes and be under the gun for the nearly 50 diseases associated with obesity. The kid touched something deep inside of me that day. As the years went on, I occasionally ran into other "Little Garys" out there, and I went out of my way to treat them with a little extra respect and compassion. With each overweight kid I ran into, I understood a little more about my own life and why everything sort of happened the way it did for me. I began to understand why my daily existence was different than other kids' and why I really never had the chance to achieve balance the way most young people did. I realized why my high school and college years were always so stilted and directionless, and how my weight negatively affected my self-esteem. I also realized why I became angry and tortured as a young man and why so many people I came into contact with always treated me as if there was something deeply wrong with me. I also began to understand why my sense of humor was always in overdrive and how I used it as a coping mechanism at an early age. With each overweight kid I spent time with, I made a little more sense of the life I had led. I would pray to God that they would figure it out before they became too old to lead normal lives. I hoped that they would never,

ever turn out like me. But with each "Little Gary," I also learned a little more about forgiveness. Like the wheelchair-bound paraplegic who accepts his predicament, with the help of these kids I was at peace with myself and with the challenge I'd been given. Life is about playing the best hand you possibly can with the cards you are dealt. Back in the winter of the new millennium, however, I was just beginning to figure all of this out.

397

In January of 2000 my wife Julie and I returned home after three weeks in Maui. In an effort to rid myself of this disease once and for all, I decided to drop in on my friend John Cannava. John had been my nutritionist early on, during my Weight Loss Clinic days. By this time he had opened his own weight loss company down the street from my office called "Metabolic Designs." I figured it was time to jump on the scale (It had literally been years) to assess what the damage was. The damage was big. *397 pounds!* As best as I can remember, the following thoughts are what raced through my mind as I watched the numbers total 397.

397...I'm in shock. I can't believe what the scale says. **397**...Oh my God! I'm a prime rib away from 400. **397**...The scale doesn't lie, especially the expensive digital model I'm on right now. **397**...I can't really be 397 pounds. **397**...This thing is killing me Elvis style. **397**...Wait a minute, how close are we to April Fools Day? **397**...At least I can feel good that I never actually reached 400 pounds. **397**...Not hitting 400 pounds is hardly an accomplishment. **397**...It doesn't get any easier if I repeat that number frequently. **397**...I don't think I look a pound over 350. **397**...Has my life really come down to this? **397**...Maybe I overdid it too much at lunch **397**...Perhaps I should strip down to my birthday suit and reweigh myself. Then again if I really weigh 397 pounds, maybe I should keep my clothes on. **397**...I've not done well. **397**...Maybe this will get me on Oprah. **397**...I don't want to be on Oprah. That's for people too heavy to get out of bed. **397**...I get out of bed no problem, at 11:00 a.m. **397**...What the hell happened in my life that I got this big? **397**...They'll have to start showering me in the car wash. **397**...They'll hook my leg up to that track and run me through on "exterior wash" **397**...Do I have a suit that fits me in case my family wants an open casket? **397**...No matter how many times I say it, it still doesn't seem real. **397**...Can I sue Weight Watchers? **397**...Perhaps I really do have a weight problem. **397**...Should I start playing those numbers in the lottery? **397**...Do I have enough money in the bank to keep my wife comfortable after my funeral and burial is paid off? **397**...How do Japanese Sumo wrestlers manage to live so long? **397**...I can't believe I'm ending my life on such a lame note. **397**…When is my next high school reunion? **397**…When I suck my stomach in and tighten my neck muscles I don't look a pound over, well, 397. **397**…Which one of my friends will try to date my wife when I'm gone? **397**…Ma's gonna be pissed. **397**…I'm never telling anyone that I actually weighed 397. **397**…What's the capacity of the average elevator? **397**…Did I really eat that much? **397**…John Belushi was only 230 when he died, so I guess I should feel lucky. **397**…I'm gonna stand here until the numbers are less than 397. **397**…How many of my friends will it take to carry my casket? **397**…Do I have enough friends? **397**…Perhaps if I change my footing the scale will actually read less than 397. **397**…There's nothing wrong with my footing. **397**…3 + 9 + 7=19, the age I wish I could return to right now. Back then I was only 297 **397**…Oh my God! I've actually been super-sized. **397**…I'll bet if I jump on another scale I'm less than 397. **397**…This is the only scale in a 60-mile radius that can handle me. **397**…How much money should I leave my nieces & nephew? **397**…I can't see a thing without my glasses. Does that say 397? **397**…Time to take a long hard look in the mirror. **397**…Rumors of my death have been greatly exaggerated…**397**…I'm gonna turn this thing around once and for all. **397**…Now about that look in the mirror.

YOU KNOW IT'S TIME TO LOSE WEIGHT WHEN...

Spring 1996: I take a client out for dinner at a restaurant near the office. "I hear the food is really good here," I tell my client. When we walk in, I'm greeted by the hostess with a hug, the bartender with a kiss, and a waiter who asks, "The pork chops again tonight for you?" It's literally like I've walked into the bar on the sitcom "Cheers." Everyone knows my name.

Halloween 1997: I go to a costume party dressed as John Popper from the Band "Blues Traveler." There aren't a lot of options for the big guys out there in terms of traditional costumes, so I buy my studded cowboy hat, harmonica, vest, sun glasses—the whole Blues Traveler look, complete with long sideburns, compliments of my wife. The problem? Nobody should have to go to a costume party dressed as a notoriously obese musician.

Summer 1995: Sitting on the deck at my uncle's Cape Cod beach house, I crash a plastic chaise lounge to the floor in five seconds flat, leaving it splintered in a million pieces on the deck. Luckily, I'm skilled at this sort of thing by now. I stop, drop and roll like a pro before the splinters of plastic can skewer me like a shish kabob. When questioned, I embarrassingly blame the implosion of the chair on the faulty 'O rings.' Twenty minutes later I'm at the mall, purchasing a replacement as well as a backup to keep in the trunk of my car, just in case.

Spring 1993: While honeymooning in Marco Island, Florida, my wife and I dine out at a restaurant on the water. It's one of those places that writes all of its nightly specials on chalkboards in the lobby. I am not initially impressed with what is on the boards and for a split second I actually consider writing in my own specials.

Christmas 1996: I receive as a gift a shirt named "Everest" from a store called "The Stout Man's Shop." The tag contains more X's than a book about Malcolm X.

Fall 1997: The local Chinese restaurant that deals in take-out only actually phones my office unsolicited to see if I might want to place an order. Is business that slow for these folks, or have I somehow become some sort of corporate account with these people? Talk about telemarketing!

Summer 1994: I accidentally set off my neighbor's smoke alarms next door by barbecuing steaks on the grill...at 10:30 pm.

Winter 1998: I'm consistently ordering an entree at restaurants with a second entree "on the side." Just to make myself feel better, I give away the side orders that accompany the second entree. That way it cancels out as an official second entree. My friends are agog.

Fall 1999: I'm cooking nightly, using the world-famous George Forman Grill. It's angled design helps the fat and oils in the cheeseburgers drain into a small tray underneath the grill itself. As soon as my twin 8 oz. burgers are done, I actually take the tray out and pour the fat and oils back onto the meat, back in their rightful place, in my mind.

Winter 2000: I order a tuxedo from the local tux shop. After giving my measurements of 60" waist and 24" neck, I overhear a voice in the background of the phone respond, "Wow, that's out there!" Thanks.

PART II
MAN ON A MISSION

ASSEMBLING YOUR WEIGHT LOSS DREAM TEAM

With the dawn of the new millennium, a new wave of quick-fix diets came on the scene and Americans quickly jumped on the wagon. Atkins. Carb Blockers. The South Beach Diet. I gave each a fleeting look and decided that I would not start yet another decade laboring away at fad diets that were unproven, and in the opinion of most experts designed to fail. I took the high road that winter and decided to dissect myself for the first time in my life.

I can't say that recruiting a team of experts to help me get healthy was the first thing I thought to do when I made the decision to take on my lifelong struggle with obesity and food addiction. But it worked out that way, and in retrospect, it was the best move I could have made. At this point I had spent nearly twenty years trying to lose weight and fix myself without ever really knowing why I was overweight in the first place. In my opinion, the absence of this knowledge is what is wrong with the weight loss industry in general. Everything is a quick-fix for a quick buck and no one is scrutinizing what the deep-seated problems might be.

By assembling a dream team of experts who specialize in all aspects of losing weight, you'll obtain the five key things you'll need to move forward and reinvent your life: education, mental conditioning, physical conditioning, accountability (to yourself and others) and focus to keep your resolve strong and your weight loss goals on track. Carefully choose each member of your team and don't be afraid to move on if someone is not working for you. You may have to go through a lot of people before you settle on what may be the most important group of people you'll ever convene in your life. Be sure your experts are bright, seasoned, and on the cutting edge of the weight loss issue. My advice is to go for the best that there is out there. Focused, sensitive, dedicated, professional and positive. They will lead you to a healing path.

MELINDA VATTURO—R.D./Nutritionist

In the winter of 2000, I decided to begin looking for a good nutritionist—someone who could reset the meter for me, start to analyze my problem, and guide me to my goal of lasting health. Julie and I were having dinner with one of our disc jockey clients one Friday night and he brought along his fiancée, Melinda. She was sweet, confident and in phenomenal shape. Now I'm no expert, but I think "hard body" would describe her best. We'd gotten together back in my hometown of Medford at my old alma mater, the Happy Haddock. By this time the place had been renamed Ruggieri's and it had gone through quite a facelift since my days working there (and I use the term "working" loosely). Aside from the infamous marinated steak tips, they now served Italian and Mexican specialties in addition to their signature seafood dishes. 20 years later, their food still took me from zero to hungry in 3.5 seconds. When it came time to order, I was engaged in a conversation with Melinda about my work. As I turned to the waitress to order my usual marinated steak tip & chicken wing combo dinner, I asked Melinda what she did for a living. "I'm a nutritionist," she answered.

"I'll have the garden salad with low-cal fat-free dressing," I told the waitress. How quickly I had plea-bargained down from a meat combo platter to a salad. We all had a laugh and went on to have a very nice dinner. The thing I liked about Melinda that night was that she never pushed the nutritionist thing. She never asked me about my weight problem (even though I was a dietitian's dream) or even talked about her work. All too often in my life I would end up sitting next to some Richard Simmons wanna-be, or Jenny Craig know-it-all-but-never-gonna-be—the "Let me tell you how I will architect a new life for you" types who just love to hear themselves talk.

I asked for Melinda's card and made an appointment to see her a month or so later. "Why a month?" you ask. Well, at this point I was not going to undertake another weight loss attempt until I knew I was deeply committed to seeing it through to it's conclusion. I had already paid the price of multiple failed diets. Lose 15, gain 30, lose the 30, gain 60, lose 60, gain 120, lose the 120 and we're into a whole new stratosphere. I'm what the medical experts call "morbidly obese." Two great words, right? It's like they've got me dead already.

At any rate, my first meeting at Melinda's office was an eye opener. Naturally, it felt good after ten years to be trying something again. But at the meeting she gave me no literature and prescribed no diet plan. The real kicker was that she never even put me on the scale. Not exactly what we think of when we think of a nutritionist, right? Then again, that kind of deja vu probably would have sent me packing and she knew it. Smart girl.

Instead, Melinda asked me for my story—my entire disparaging history dealing with food addiction, weight gain and weight loss. What diets I had tried at what ages. What my family's attitudes and approaches were. She explored what my eating habits had been at various stages of my life and what food environments I'd been in. The whole sorry deal. Melinda explained to me that my problem was extremely complex and most likely not due to any one particular factor. There were probably five or six different factors that caused me to be overweight in the first place. She explained that together as a team we would have to step back and break down each one of these factors and deal with them individually. In my case, she felt there was probably heredity, emotional eating, bad habits, psychological issues, a slow metabolism, and complete lack of exercise. Dissect each of these factors; carefully develop strategies for dealing with each one, and you're on your way. The first thing Melinda asked me to do was visualize what I wanted my healthy body to look like. "You'll see it when you believe it," as my friend Tom Hayes has said.

Secondly, she asked me to keep a daily journal. Yes that's right, the "food journal" thing. We've all heard that one before. In this case, however, it wasn't so Melinda could track what I was eating and correct me like some tightly-wound schoolteacher. I would later learn it was for my own personal accountability. Psychologically, it had an immediate impact on me. It opened my eyes to the huge amount of food I was actually consuming each day. Talk about continuing to pump gas into a car when the tank is full! I needed a "No Topping Off" sign around my waist. Almost immediately, I began backing off on the frequency and amount of what I was eating. The power of positive journaling grew as time went on. Eventually, I recorded my emotions, what I was feeling, and what the circumstances were when I overate. This was incredibly helpful in dissecting myself.

There was a third thing Melinda asked me to try, which was eating with the clock. Breakfast religiously at 8:00 a.m. every morning. Lunch at noon sharp. Dinner no later than 6:00 p.m. Almost immediately, the addict-like cravings disappeared and the hunger pangs became a distant memory. That powerful inner impulse to eat that most food addicts experience suddenly subsided, and if nothing else, was under control. Amazing, yet so simple, and it truly made a world of difference. I realized that eating with the clock was a healthy habit for life and a significant step towards defeating food addiction. People who have successfully lost the weight and kept it off will always tell you it is like learning how to ride a bike. Learn how to eat with the clock and you're ready to remove the training wheels and move on to the next phase.

To my bafflement, my initial weight loss was very slow in coming, but Melinda was shrewdly focusing on important factors beyond the raw numbers on the scale. She dissected my strong connection to food and evaluated my addiction. She also began the long and complicated process of identifying what had been damaged by my addiction: namely, my sense of self-restraint. After all, at the end of the day, who made you eat pizza in the middle of the night? In those moments where you make the decision to abuse food, you can blame it on your addiction, but in the end, the decision to act on that impulse is really between you and yourself.

The complexities of my food issues were amazing to me. There seemed to be multiple levels and long-time habits to determine. The snails pace of my weight loss suggested that my metabolism had taken a serious hit from all the years of perennial dieting.

As the summer of 2000 dragged on, Melinda began to notice how psychological my food issues were. Frankly, I think I may have taxed the poor girl. Perhaps we were getting into an area beyond her expertise. Maybe she just didn't have all day to listen to my rants about my weight loss battle. At any rate, she recommended a friend of hers who was a clinical social worker and therapist who specialized in weight issues. Dream team member number two, come on down!

RUTH SCHWARTZ, LICSW, CAS

I was lying pool-side when I called Ruth from my cell phone on a 90-degree day in August. What better time to get motivated to call? It was summer and there I was, dressed like I was at a toga party. There was an extra large bath sheet wrapped around me and a towel around my neck. I hadn't been in the pool yet because I was waiting for the two or three people swimming in the pool to leave. I refused to be fodder for their dinnertime conversations. I made an appointment with Ruth at her home office instead of her work office. The home office had the comfy couch. Let's face it, it's all about the couch. Ruth was everything I hoped she would be. Fifty-something, eyeglass-wearing CNN-psychology-expert-correspondent type. Intelligent, educated, polished, brutally honest, and at times like a long lost mother. I'd been missing my own so badly and Ruth captured Rainbow's sweet well-meaning demeanor, probably more than she realized. She also had Rainbow's stern "now why would you ever say a thing like that about yourself?" attitude. Refreshing when you are a racecar stuck in first gear.

I'm not sure if Ruth was fascinated or horrified by me the first time we met. All I know is that I lay there horizontal for 50 minutes, talking about my thoughts on health, life and my need to acquire both. Her eyebrows slowly raised above her glasses and stayed glued there as I went on and on about my weight, my career, mental health, marriage, family, etc.

"How did it go?" asked Julie when I walked through the door that night.

"Good, I guess. She wants me to come back tomorrow," I responded.

Julie looked confused. "Tomorrow?" she asked. Who could blame my wife for being surprised? Who ever heard of someone going back to a therapist the very next day? Hardly normal. Let's face it, either Ruth Schwartz had an opening she wanted to fill or I was a powerful lesson in human imperfection. Truthfully, I didn't really want to know the answer, but I went back the next day, and roughly twice monthly after that.

With Ruth on the Dream Team, I had answers to questions I'd contemplated for years and years. She helped me identify the origins of my addiction and how my upbringing had impacted the problem. She showed me how anxiety and stress played such a key role in the addiction and how to avoid putting myself in "perverse atmospheres" in the future. She emphasized the importance of finding things in life beyond food that could give me the same pleasure and how to take stock of things that had not been negatively affected by my food issues. Ruth shot holes in my "life is a bust" attitude and helped me appreciate the positive things in my life. She taught me to see the Pu Pu Platter as half full, if you will. All of this wisdom for a ten-dollar co-payment? Now if you're a bargain shopper, you can't do much better than that, can you?

She also confirmed for me some of my thoughts on the whole health/weight mess. How much off-course we'd gotten in terms of our portion sizes. How wrong 90% of the weight loss companies were in their approaches! Ruth stressed again and again the importance of accepting my overeating as a disease. "It's an addiction, Gary," she would say in an attempt to stifle my frustrations. At first I honestly had a hard time accepting that I was an actual food addict. Drug and Alcohol addiction is one thing, but to stare at a plate of Buffalo wings and admit that you have no control? That would take a little time. As I began focusing on my actions and feelings while in the presence of food, I had to concede that the connection was very similar to that of the alcoholics I've known in my life.

When I first began seeing Ruth, I expressed my frustration over how much weight I had to lose and communicated my doubts that I could actually ever get to a goal weight.

"You will," she answered confidently, with a tone of wisdom in her voice. "Over the course of the next two to three years, Gary, you'll slowly learn to de-emphasize food and its importance in your life, and you will lose the weight."

Exactly the words I didn't want to hear. You see, at this point I was still all about the "quick fix." I think most Americans are. We want to lose the weight fast so we can get back to the business of eating the foods we love, then we con ourselves into thinking we somehow will remain fit and healthy at the same time. We all have that fantasy, and we all have to be resigned to the fact that it's just that: a fantasy. The reality is that it's a long process to reprogram your eating and recondition your exercising habits. If you've yo-yo dieted your entire life and destroyed your metabolism like I have, the process is going to be that much harder. The good news is that we all have the opportunity to do it—if we choose to. In the end, what's two or three years as long as you get there?

As time went on, Ruth's words became strikingly true. They resonate with me even to this day. Between my biweekly visits with both Melinda and Ruth, my road to recovery began to take on a life of its own. With the information I gleaned from our meetings, I became more and more fascinated with learning about health. The questions were basic, but important: where I had been, and more importantly, where I was going. Like a private eye conducting a grand investigation, I found myself digging and digging for more knowledge. I'll even go so far as to say it became "intoxicating" to learn about the mental and physical aspects of getting healthy. Not bad for a guy who just five months earlier was dipping bread into BBQ sauce after polishing off two racks of ribs in Hawaii. My unquenchable thirst for information and knowledge rivaled my one-time thirst for strawberry ice cream shakes. The more information I sought out, the more experts I added to my Dream Team.

DR. BERTRAM ZARINS, M.D., F.A.C.S
Chief of Sports Medicine, Massachusetts General Hospital

Bertram Zarins has long been considered one of the top sports medicine doctors in the world. He's been the team physician for the Boston Bruins and the New England Patriots for many years, as well as a council member for the U.S. Olympic Sports Committee. At Massachusetts General Hospital he is highly esteemed and widely regarded as being one of the best in the industry. When New England Patriot's star quarterback, Drew Bledsoe, developed potentially career-ending knee injuries, it was Zarins who guided him back to health and eventually to that memorable 2002 Super Bowl Season. Now I'm sure a 400-pound, Hawaiian-shirted food addict from Medford MA was hardly on Zarins' A-List, but thanks to my primary care physician, Dr. Jeffrey Harris, I managed to get an appointment.

Harris recommended Zarins after I had complained of ankle and foot pain during a routine physical. At this point, I'd just begun walking five to six miles per day and knew little about the sport of power walking. Well, I'd walked more than my share of mall food courts, but this was something new. Harris was impressed that I was attempting to turn my health around with an aggressive walking and exercise routine every day, so he recommended Zarins because of his work with the Patriots. "He specializes in big guys who put huge physical stress on their bodies, not unlike you," he said. Now I was hardly in New England Patriots shape, but I knew what he was talking about. There weren't a heck of a lot of people out there distance-walking every day that looked like me. I knew that if I injured myself exercising the wrong way, a huge part of my recovery would be interrupted, possibly permanently. Exercise and eating right. Eating right and exercise. The two go hand in hand.

I decided that if Zarins would have me, I would put him in light rotation on the Dream Team's schedule. Dr. Zarins was great. He was a tall, handsome guy who wore a Hollywood smile at all times. He wasted no time in assessing my situation, giving me solid advice, and writing a prescription for special support socks. The socks would keep my ankles lined up correctly mile after mile. I was amazed at how complex and scientific my exercise of choice was. Every bone and muscle was connected to something else.

Dr. Zarins and his staff were skilled, professional, and incredibly helpful. From them I learned I had a condition known as "Supination," which affects many runners and walkers. To supinate is to habitually walk on the sides of the feet, which results in painful burning sensations on the outside bands of the legs. "It sounds like it could also result in a burning sensation in one's wallet from purchasing new sneakers every month," I joked with Zarins' staff.

I surmised that if I had to experience burning sensations somewhere in my body, the outside of the legs was not the worst place, but Dr. Zarins' staff thought it could become a problem with the mileage I planned to do. The fact was, I already had been waking up several times a night with extreme pain on the sides of my legs. The condition could only get worse and would not necessarily go away with my weight loss. I had also been averaging a pair of sneakers every month because the sides wore down from the supination. They explained to me that many Boston Marathon runners suffered from the same condition, so Dr. Zarins' office wrote me a second prescription for 1/3" angled inserts for my sneakers. The inserts leveled out my feet and kept the situation under control. They also encouraged me to alternate my mileage every day. They penned out a sample schedule of six miles on Monday, four on Tuesday, three on Wednesday, five on Thursday, and so on. This, they explained, would reduce the wear and tear on my feet as well.

By the end of 2000, the initial members of my Dream Team were in place. I planned to add other people, such as fitness trainers, once I had had some initial success. With all of the solid advice and conditioning orbiting my mind and body almost daily, I felt poised to achieve true health and happiness for the first time in years. I had, as you can tell, nowhere else to go but down, either to an early grave, or to a lesser weight. I chose the road less traveled. With the help of Melinda, Ruth, Dr. Zarins and others, I headed out on that road and never looked back.

DISSECTING THE DISORDER

For years I had searched for the answer to one simple question: what would it take to push my inner button and finally lose the weight? How much abuse, mental anguish and self-torture would one guy have to go through before he woke up with the resolve to finally get healthy? How many years would go by before he could step off the "if only I could lose a few pounds" roller coaster?

I knew that if I could answer that question I could not only achieve true health, but also help countless other food addicts like myself. Somehow, that would justify everything I'd been through. If I could light the fire under even one person besides myself, I could come to terms with the years I'd spent as a hopeless food addict, seemingly stuck in self-destruct mode.

The truth is, the answer that I so desperately sought was right in front of me all the time. What finally pushed my inner button was not one more insult on the street, one more failed relationship, or one more crashed piece of furniture. It was much simpler than that. It was the actual process of dissecting the disorder—agreeing with myself not to ignore it any longer, nor to accept it any longer, facing myself every day and acknowledging what my life had become and would continue to be as long as I had this chocolate chip on my shoulder. or the first time in my life, I decided to admit the complexity of my problem. No hiding my weight with over-sized, over-priced outfits. I wasn't a rap star. No more pretending my weight problem did not have far-reaching effects and no more staying away from the things I'd always wanted to do in life.

Dissecting the disorder is the blueprint to changing what's really staring back at you in the mirror. As I've previously mentioned, Melinda prescribed no exercise and designed no diet plan on that first meeting. Instead, she talked about the complexity of my problem, led me to that very important blueprint, and described how it would be necessary to step back and break down every bad habit, negative cycle, food craving and genetic trait by keeping food journals every day. Not for her, but for me. Breaking down my impulse to eat into little dissected bits of information helped me make sense of my longtime disorder. What was I feeling during the cravings? Was I even hungry? What had I eaten previously? How did it affect me? What food really was good for me and what was simply advertised to be? I broke it all down and this process, in itself, actually pushed my inner button. Who knew that such a simple thing would be the key to pushing the inner button? The more I studied nutrition, exercise, the human body and the environmental factors that led to 61% of the country being over-weight at the time, the more I understood how human I actually was. This was not as powerful a problem as I'd always believed it was. It *could be* dealt with and eventually conquered. Dissecting my entire approach to everything I ate was the mental conditioning that put me on the right track. Once I'd fully faced my food connection head on and begun studying it, I was ready to get going on the next part of the equation: getting educated.

In August of 2001 I heard about a full-day seminar on food cravings that was tak-ing place at the Sheraton Hotel in Lexington, MA. The cost was $80.00 for the full day. *Sign me up. Life's too short to live like this.*

At 8:00 a.m. the instructor put up the opening PowerPoint slide. It read, "Just because you have a craving, doesn't mean you have to act on it." To me that was a mind-blowing and brilliant concept. Stop the presses! So when I have a craving and attempt to fulfill it I don't actually have to act on it? Wow! What a simple, yet insightful, concept. That's probably the first thing out of every weight loss specialist's mouth. At 8:00 in the morning I had already gotten my $80.00 worth. I didn't *have* to go racing for the drive-through every time I had a craving for a burger. If I waited 10-20 minutes or concentrated on other things, the crav-ings would pass. It's a scientific fact. It only took me 35 years to figure that one out. The truth of the matter was that by the time I came across this terrific advice, my cravings had dropped off significantly already. A year before, Melinda had convinced me to eat with the clock. Again, so simple, and yet it made all the dif-ference in the world. By consistently eating at 8:00 a.m., noon, and 6:00 p.m., 80% of my cravings were suddenly gone. I began to realize that they were simply the result of bad eating habits. Skip breakfast and you'll crave unhealthy food by 10:30 a.m. Eat dinner late and you'll skip breakfast the next morning because you are still full. 10:30 a.m. would come and I'd be craving Chinese food. We're talking sweet & sour chicken at 10:00 in the morning, folks! And it would hap-pen again tomorrow if I skipped breakfast.

After the seminar, I began to realize that I was not so much a severe food addict as I was a lover of food whose bad eating patterns had caused addict-like cravings. Control those bad habits and you'll be officially downgraded from hopeless food addict to hopeful food enthusiast. Food sportsman, professional food technician, whatever title you want to give it, it's a major improvement and very empowering. The mere fact that I was attending a food-craving seminar was every bit as important as what was learned in the seminar. The inner button had been pushed, and just when it seemed like I had dissected myself enough, something new would come up that would force me to take a closer look at situations, bad habits or temptations. I'll never declare victory over this disorder, but if I continue to study myself I'll be able to control it. In a very important way, that will always be a major victory.

I learned another important part of the dissecting process in one of my sessions with Ruth Schwartz, who was by now one of my favorite people. Ruth taught me to identify perverse atmospheres I should avoid while I try to lose weight. Initially, the term "perverse atmosphere" conjured up memories of Pee Wee Herman walking into an adult movie theater. However, the double entendre aside, it actually made sense. An addict is an addict. Now, I'm not trying to discourage people caught in the weight loss struggle from eating in these particular establishments. I'm just trying to demonstrate that perverse atmospheres exist in everyone's life and in every town in the USA.

WARNING: SKIPPING THIS PORTION OF THE CHAPTER CAN GREATLY REDUCE YOUR TEMPTATION TO HEAD FOR A REFRIGERATOR NEAR YOU...

Top 5 Perverse Places to be in if you are me:

(1) Hungry Herb's, Medford, MA

Hands down, Herb's is the mother of all sub joints. You know the one in your town where the steak tips are piled so high on the bulkie roll that you have to eat the entire meal with a fork? Where the BBQ sauce soaks down the roll, rendering it useless? That's Herb's place. The sandwiches come in two sizes: The Herb (large) and Herbie (small). The problem is, for those of us watching our weight, the Herbie isn't really that small at all. Teriyaki chicken tips. Honey mustard and sweet BBQ turkey tips. Cajun anything. Buffalo chicken tips that can send your sinus infections running for the door. Steak fries the size of your big toe and chili so thick and tasty you'll swear they shipped it in right from Texas. Herb himself is a tall, friendly, teddy bear of a man whose famous saying is, "Nice." When you place your order with Herb, the conversation usually sounds something like this.

HERB: Can I help you, young man?

Me: Sure, Herb. I'll have the Ginger and Honey BBQ Turkey Tips.

HERB: Nice!

Me: And a side of the Chili, with extra Cheddar Cheese.

HERB: Niiiccceee…

Me: And how about an extra large order of the potato skins with sour cream and bacon bits?

HERB: Nice, nice! And what to wash that down with, my good friend?

Me: Let's do a 30 oz. Coke.

HERB: Very niiiccceee, young man! That will be up in about ten minutes.

Simply put, if you're not all wrapped up in the health thing, don't miss this place if you're passing through town. Unfortunately, for me it's not so "nice."

(2) Kowloon Restaurant, Saugus, MA

Standing on the outside of this massive structure on US Route 1 North, you'll swear you're in Tiananmen Square. What you will actually be standing outside of is the number one grossing Chinese restaurant in the continental United States, and I know why. It's worth it! Boneless pork ribs? They speak to me. Fresh crab rangoon and Kowloon special fried rice? It's almost sexual. Chinese lobster smothered in butter and garlic? I think I've just met the Lord. Just walking into this place these days puts me on heightened alert. Trust me, the well-endowed egg rolls and Szechwan and Polynesian dishes are right on so many levels, and yet if you're a food addict like me, it's all so wrong.

(3) MIKE'S DONUT SHOP, Everett, MA

My God, do I have a tough time driving past Mike's! Hands down, it's the Disney World of donut places. A Hollywood movie about Mike's would be titled, "Honey, I blew up the pastry!" Fresh Apple Crumb and Vanilla Crème Donuts the size of a bean bag chair. You bite into one side and filling the size of your fist shoots out the other, so dress appropriately. Polish off more than two of their famous Coconut Custard Donuts and head for your primary care physician because you'll want to have a diabetes test. Who says donuts have to be warm and "Krispy?" And as if Mike's Donut Shop isn't over the top enough, they have actually had the nerve to add calzones to their repertoire: Italian, meatball, steak, and cheese. For folks not suffering from my disease, I suggest you back the car up, pop the trunk, and load up on everything at Mike's. A dozen for the car and a dozen for the house! Me? I'll be avoiding this end of town altogether.

(4) Chianti Restaurant, Beverly, MA

Okay, I've got to throw in a plug for my brother Richard here. Leave it to me to have a relative who happens to own one of the most outrageous gourmet Italian restaurants in the New England area. Lobster ravioli, pumpkin tortellini, roasted butternut squash pasta oozing with garlic flavor. And for dessert, how about an order of crème brulée or a hunk of tiramisu, my brother's personal recipe? It even hurts to write about it, but lucky for me by 2003 that creative brother of mine was close to doing the unthinkable. He began working on creating healthy, low-calorie, low-carbohydrate gourmet Italian dishes. Godspeed, my brother, Godspeed!

(5) Kings Grant Inn—Danvers, MA

I went to a Sunday brunch buffet here back in 1987 with the entire family. I swear I've never been the same since. Custom-made omelets heaped with ham, mushrooms, onions and assorted cheeses. Fresh Belgian Waffles with waves of maple syrup, strawberries and whipped cream. Stop the madness, people! Bacon, ham, corned beef hash, home fried potatoes, mountains of Kielbasa and sausages, fresh muffins, crepes, bagels and pastry, that whole carbohydrate overdose we see everywhere these days. And just in case your breakfast time overflows into lunch, there are plenty of non-breakfast items: beef and pork ribs, lasagna, fish casseroles, fresh carved meats, mashed potatoes, baked potatoes, and potatoed potatoes. Talk about a theme park for food addicts! Finally, just in case you've inhaled too much food, Kings Grant happens to be an Inn! Do what I did, and use your Visa card to rent a room so you can recover from your chowfest on the premises. Luckily, Kings Grant was sold for office space in 2003. For me, there is a God.

(6) Michelbob's Ribs, Naples, FL

I know I said this was going to be my Top 5 perverse atmospheres, but I would simply be lying if I left this place off my list. Michelbob's Ribs is a two-time winner of the "Best Ribs in America" award and the current "World's Best Sauce" defending champion. Did you even know they had awards for this stuff? More importantly, from what I can tell they're only getting better. Massive racks of tasty pork and beef ribs. The meat falls off the bone and into your mouth. Just in case there's not enough barbecue sauce on the ribs when they arrive, there are bottles of assorted sauces on every table. Do you want the sweet or the tangy? How about both? You can never be too sure in these troubled times, can you? You'll need more than a few moist towelettes when you're done, so grab about 30 or so. Better yet, do what I used to do. Wear junky clothes that you can throw away when you're finished or have a friend hose you off out back.

On our honeymoon back in 1993, Julie snapped pictures of me in front of the "Michelbob's Ribs" sign and in the kitchen with the chef who prepared the ribs. In the photos I resembled a kid meeting Mickey Mouse for the very first time. *Gary Marino, you just won two free plane tickets to anywhere in the world. Where are you gonna go? I'm going to Michelbob's!*

◆   ◆   ◆

By September 2001, despite the existence of such perverse atmospheres, I had been eating healthy and walking up a storm. Like Forrest Gump on steroids, you could find me on any given day miles off the beaten track, walking or hiking in the woods. I was on fire and on my game, but perplexed as to why I wasn't losing a lot of weight. I scheduled a session with Melinda and started off with the line, "We've got to check for a thyroid problem; the weight is just not coming off the way it should." I'll bet she has heard that line more than once or twice. We all are, unfortunately, prone to denial on what we put into our mouths. We are also conditioned to believe that the way we've eaten all our lives is somehow normal.

"I've done a complete turnaround in what I eat and the exercise that I get, yet the weight is coming off painfully slowly," I told her.

"Let's have a closer look at what you're eating these days," she responded very calmly, with a hint of *I know the answer without looking* in her voice. I followed her into a nearby conference room to look at my carefully kept food records. This is where dissecting becomes key.

"For starters, let's look at the fruit you're consuming," she said. "Orange juice in the morning, pineapple chunks as a mid-morning snack, grapes in your salads, and bananas in your cereal. Too much fruit." Initially I was surprised, because like many overweight Americans, I believed that "too much fruit" could never be a negative to one's diet. But what Melinda pointed out made sense. All those fruits and all those sugars certainly amounted to something. "Sugars are carbohydrates," she reminded me. Next up on the "too much" list was yogurt. "I like the fact that you're getting calcium," she said, "but two to three cups of vanilla flavored yogurt with sliced strawberries is again too much." Now it was beginning to make sense. An overdose of healthy food is still an overdose. Melinda had never actually given me a specific number of calories to consume daily (part of her overall strategy to keep me from feeling policed), but the numbers on the scale were a clear indicator that I was still taking in too many. "Cut back to three fruit servings per day and cut your cereal intake down from two cups to one," she suggested. Other foods I was consuming in my new era of health included energy bars and protein products. They were being advertised constantly, and the stores were beginning to stock entire aisles dedicated to meal replacement bars. Although they were better than your average candy bar, most were still filled with corn syrup, coco butter, sugars, carbohydrates, sodium, sucrose, fructose, mononitrate, and "Mambo Number 5." You get the picture. Whatever they were advertised as, they were at best a healthy candy bar, and I was eating at least one a day. In an attempt to realign my food intake, Melinda scratched protein bars off my list as well as a few other items. She gave me other tips as well. "Try soy milk instead of regular milk," she instructed, "and buy a kitchen scale to measure how much meat you're cooking. Keep it to six to eight ounces and buy six-packs of small yogurt servings, being sure to check the calories, carbohydrates, and sugars." By the end of the session, Melinda had pretty much come to the conclusion that although I had been eating healthy foods, it was still too much for it to amount to any substantial weight loss. "You're switching out bad calories for good calories, Gary, but keep in mind that it's still a game of calories in the end. Try to keep it to 1600 or so."

Over the period of the next two years, Melinda and I continued to dissect what I was consuming over and over and it became a fascinating process for me. We honed it. We added certain things and eliminated others. We left nothing to chance. Losing weight is a very scientific process; burn more calories than you take in. The dissecting process opened my eyes to what healthy eating truly was, and as time went on I began to hold myself more and more accountable. Study it, analyze it, and dissect it. The process itself will push your resolve to places it has never been before. I promise you'll never regret it. It will make your health goals come true.

POWER WALKING:
Don't be Careless about Calluses!

"Those long solo walks you are taking are a metaphor for your life these days. You are taking control of your life for the first time. Things are going to change incredibly for you now because it means you will be taking control of your health, personal relationships and business dealings. Many of the people around you will not adjust well to what you are doing for yourself. The road can be lonely, much like those walks, but out of this you will emerge from this a better, stronger and happier person..."

—Dr. Lillian Arleque, motivational speaker and lifecoach

So at what point did Powerwalking become an actual sport? For me, I guess it became a sport the day I finally succumbed to the fact that I'd have to do some form of exercise every day for the rest of my life. The day I accepted that fact, I was on my way.

Like most overweight people, I'd spent most of my life fantasizing that I could actually lose the weight and look great without any exercise whatsoever. Dieting was enough of a sacrifice and exercise was a drag, in my opinion. Deep down, of course, I knew that one without the other was fruitless. Melinda's philosophy of 75% in favor of exercise vs. the usual 50/50 made sense. I decided that aggressive walking, in conjunction with the food plan that Melinda and I had agreed on, would be my 75%/25% health equation. I also promised myself that once I achieved a certain degree of weight loss I would incorporate traditional sports into my life, such as tennis, basketball, swimming and weight training.

In the past I'd tried power walking and actually liked it, but as soon as my diets had failed, the exercise was as good as dead. Sometimes the process had worked in reverse. I developed calluses or injuries to my ankles first, then with my exercise routine sidelined, I'd fall off whatever program I was on. This time I had no intention of failing. It was time to get healthy once and for all. I decided that if I was going to get aggressive about walking, I'd best get educated on issues such as proper footwear. In addition to the supination, I'd been cursed with extra wide feet (size 6E in width), to go with everything else that was wide. The first thing I did was get a recommendation from one of Dr. Zarins' assistants for sneakers. The assistant suggested Runner's Edge in Melrose, MA, which served many of the runners in the Boston Marathon each year. I got there on a Wednesday night just before closing time, and a nice sales guy named Tony Pallotta immediately asked me if I needed help. "I'm looking for some good walking sneakers," I told him.

"Okay," Tony responded. "Where do you do most of your walking?"

"Well, mostly Memory Lane the last 10 years or so, but it doesn't burn many calories," I joked. (Don't worry, Tony didn't get it either). He then immediately asked me to get on a treadmill in the back of the store.

"Geez, I know I need to lose weight, but isn't this a bit much?" I asked. Tony laughed and explained that the reason he needed me to walk the treadmill was so he could videotape my walk and determine how severe my supination was. If my condition was not dealt with correctly, my walking could be stopped in its tracks for weeks. That would slow the process down and hurt my overall resolve. After taping me on the treadmill, Tony studied the tape and suggested a model called "The Beast." *Here we go with the names again*, I thought. *A guy could get a complex, you know?* I purchased two pairs of "The Beast" and two pairs of New Balance Motion Control Walkers just to balance the support on my feet. From there I headed for the mall to purchase the next piece of equipment, which in my opinion was equally important: a good personal CD player. It's all about the music, isn't it, folks? It's the music that pumps you up, gets you excited, and makes you feel like Rocky Balboa climbing those steps in downtown Philadelphia. I purchased two CD players, and with the help of one of my disc jockeys, created a series of customized *Million Calorie March* CDs, designed to push my motivation to places it had never been. The CDs had different themes, such as classics, 80s, rock & roll, soul (searching) music—you name it, I had a CD to fit my every mood. One day I'd listen to Led Zep's "Good Times, Bad Times," and the next it would be Elton John's "The Simple Life."

Music wasn't the only thing I changed on a frequent basis. I switch up locations almost daily, just to keep it fresh. I was never much of a treadmill person (unless it had a TV mount and an hors d'oeuvres tray extension), but occasionally I jumped on one. I rarely walked the same walk two days in a row. It'd be the Mystic Lakes in Medford on Monday, the track at Tufts University on Tuesday, the inspirational neighborhood with the million-dollar homes on Wednesday, a beach in Cape Cod on Thursday, the reservoir at Fresh Pond in Cambridge on Friday. Saturday was when I'd head for the deep woods somewhere. We're not talking about trails and paths through a forest somewhere. We're talking about heading off the trails and into the *deep bush*. It's a bit bizarre, I know, but the kid in me loved the challenge of climbing rocks, discovering beautiful ponds in the middle of nowhere and finding hidden plateaus surrounded by nothing but thick green forest. I also loved the challenge of finding my way back through the woods. That'll keep it fresh every time and add an extra hour to the old workout, right?

My friends always gave me a hard time about walking alone in the middle of nowhere for hours on end. "Do you wear face paint when you go?" they joked. "Do you become *one with nature?*" The possibility of me getting lost always seemed to make people nervous, even though I assured them that I carried my cell phone with me. I might have been a little crazy, but I wasn't stupid.

Not very long ago a family member said in jest, "I can see this on the six o'clock news someday, 'He lived on sticks, bugs and the bark off trees for 40 weeks before crawling out of the woods on his hands and knees'. "

"Maybe so," I laughed, "but here's how the rest of the story goes. 'He took a shower, went on "Good Morning America" and hit the speaking circuit at twenty grand a pop!'

That's Big Guys 3, skeptical friend 0, if you're still keeping score at home.

ANALYZE THIS:
Revisiting your youth

"I've been thinking about getting back into shape…then I realized I've never actually been in shape…I have absolutely nothing to get back to!"

—*Comedian Tony V on NBC's Late Night with Conan O'Brien*

For years I tried to fix myself with "fad of the month" diets. Looking back, it was a pretty flawed approach. A desperate attempt to get my life back on track with the help of liquid or herbal diets, pre-packaged food diets or whatever would get me thin the fastest. I was always anxious to get it over with and get on with my reckless youth. A pretty unrealistic game plan, now that I think of it. Maybe that's human nature. Frequent dieters will know what I'm talking about here. You sign up for these programs and the first thing they tell you is why their program works better than the others and how much weight you can expect to lose. "By the way, make the check out to…" It's amazing, when I think of it. One minute you are in the waiting room looking at before & after photos, the next minute you are being given a food plan for the rest of your life. Of course I never seemed to meet any of the people in the before & after photos. Apparently they were on some weight loss relocation program somewhere, probably looking a heck of a lot like their before photos. The word "diet" is no longer around. Neither are a lot of those programs, come to think of it. A misguided effort to say the least. Nobody in 20 years tried to study my habits to see why I was overweight. Occasionally they would have me keep a journal to see how well I was sticking to their regimen, but what about the regimen that got me to a life threatening 397 pounds in the first place?

While vacationing in Hawaii in 2000, I took a long walk on the beach and thought hard about my childhood. You know, it wasn't all bad. A lot of good times were had. I had some really great memories. But the "Big Guy" thing, it was always a part of my life. There was always plenty of speculation from others about what would work for me, but no concrete answers. I realized this was important to know before I began a final attempt. By this point in my life I well understood that years of failed diets had only increased my weight. I decided I would not truly begin until I had a better understanding as to where I had been and what my approach to food had done to my health. If I could finally identify and understand the factors that made me overweight, that would be my "GO" point. The following is what I came up with.

GENETIC PREDISPOSITION

First let me say that genetics are in no way a cop-out or a crutch. I do not want sympathy delivered or excuses made for my lifelong weight problem, nor do I want to blame my entire family tree, but here are the facts. It's in the family. My mother was overweight, her brother was overweight, their parents were overweight, and my grandfather had 13 brothers & sisters, all who were overweight. When I looked at his family photos as a kid I had to chuckle, as not one person in the family was less than 250 pounds. Even the women in the family, such as his sister Concetta, looked to be around a deuce and a half. Nowadays it's not so funny. If I took half of my siblings and cousins, dressed them in 1930s clothing and used an old-fashioned black & white camera to photograph them, the pictures would be frighteningly similar. If there was ever any doubt at all that the fat gene exists in our family, the proof is in those old, fading photographs. None of this, of course, means that I have to live my life as a 400-pound individual, but it does mean that I need to work a lot harder to stay trim. Now most weight loss experts allow that the heredity factor can account for as much as 30% of an individual's weight issue. However, before you go diving for the family photo album, consider that how and where your ancestors were raised also comes into play. Who knows? Perhaps you can change the course of things for your future grandchildren by establishing a healthy lifestyle right now.

POST-TRAUMATIC STRETCH DISORDER

Like many people, I am an emotional eater. If something traumatic happens to me or if I'm under a lot of stress, I make a dash for food. Good food, bad food, drive-thru or gourmet, it doesn't matter. Food is comforting. It feels good going down, like an emotional pat on the back. It's a quick fix and unfortunately one that leads to a cycle of more stress and trauma. Emotional eating is a big part of the obesity equation. More and more studies reveal the fact that over-eating is directly linked to anxiety and stress, two words which, unfortunately, have become synonymous with the American way of life. Stress eating, emotional bingeing, post-traumatic stretch disorder, or whatever you want to label it. These actions essentially fall under the category of "bad habits" and can kill your healthy resolve for years and years. Take it from me.

OVEREMPHASIZING FOOD

As I've mentioned, both of my parents were incredible Italian cooks, which unfortunately was one of the reasons I formed a weight problem at a fairly young age. Food was definitely celebrated—a reason to get excited. In retrospect, I feel we rallied around food a little more than we should have. Holidays were over the top. There was never enough real estate on the tables and countertops to house the endless platters of food and desserts. As kids, we definitely "oohed" and "aahed" a lot around food. We probably weren't as bad as some families (we were raised more American-Italian than Italian-American), but I definitely grew up in a home where food was a big deal. Mom, I think, understood this and tried not to do what her parents had done to her, but in the end she was only human. De-emphasizing food is one of the most important things you can do for your child. Teach them that food is fuel, not love. Reward them with non-food treats literally from the time they are in the highchair. Don't serve family-style dinners—with serving bowls on the table—but prepare each plate with sensible portions. And always teach your kids to eat for their bodies instead of their taste buds.

YO-YO DIETING

On this subject, I'm textbook. Lose 20, gain 40. Lose 40, gain 80. Lose 160 and the next thing you know, you're super-sized. Losing is a big risk if the weight loss isn't permanent. You pay the price once that cycle has started. I will always maintain that had my parents not introduced me to the word "diet" at age thirteen, I would still would have gone on to have a weight problem, but nothing like the aberration I became: 230, 240, maybe 250—but 397? I doubt it. In my humble opinion, years of losing and gaining the weight exacerbated the problem beyond what it would have been. In all fairness, my folks had no idea. They were just the typical 1970s parents, trying to help me avoid a "waisted youth." Their hearts were in the right place, but unfortunately I went on to become everything they had hoped I wouldn't. I'll always regret that. Life is truly a hard road when you grow up overweight. Anyone who says it isn't is only fooling him or herself.

BAD HABITS

It doesn't take a specialist to identify bad eating habits, but ignore them or blow them off and you're ignoring a big piece of the puzzle. Everyone's bad habits are different, but in my case they ranged from not keeping healthy, readily available foods in the refrigerator to literally skipping breakfast for years and starting each day off on the wrong foot. Building my social schedule around restaurants was also a bad habit. Monday morning dieting, or waiting for the beginning of the week to eat healthy again, was another. I could go on, but why bother? Dissect yourself and you'll be amazed at how addict-like symptoms can be shown the door.

DELAYING REALITY

Growing up, I always used food and my weight problem as a device to delay reality. As far as I was concerned, I was never truly in the game of life. Staying overweight was truly a way to avoid facing the challenges in life that most kids go through. I always had doubts that the "thin Gary" who everyone pushed me to be could live up to their expectations. I believe that subconsciously I overate to avoid the challenges of being a good athlete, a good student, being good with the women, or frankly being good at anything. By maintaining a weight problem, I never had to face the truth about life or my abilities to excel at it. It was a bizarre way to grow up. No matter how much pain I went through being overweight, deep inside I was unsure that I could handle life, so the weight problem was my crutch. As I got older and more confident of my abilities, this type of self-sabotage dropped off considerably. But was it a factor in the overall problem? You betcha!

EATING FOR THE TASTEBUDS INSTEAD OF THE BODY

The cultural tradition in America. Place a bowl of Lucky Charms cereal and a cup of yogurt and almonds in front of the average American, and which one would they rather eat? With the overwhelming majority of Americans overweight, my money's on the one with the magic marshmallows. Problem is, your body gets absolutely nothing out of it but a high sugar overdose. Once I began to face my disease and learn about what the human body actually needs, I began to realize just how far off course my eating was. I'll go more into this in future chapters, but that old saying is true: food is fuel, not love!

SIGNIFICANT OTHER—SIGNIFICANT PROBLEM

When I got engaged, I was hardly a picture of health. Julie's eating habits were not a factor in my own. As long as she enjoyed fast food, late night binges, and a refrigerator jammed with fatty options, I was giving that girl a ring. Julie did not have a weight problem or a problem with mine, which, let's face it, is what every overweight guy dreams of. Years later, as I began to dissect my eating disorder, I realized just how important it is to have your wife on board 100 percent. A bad influence is a bad influence. Julie ate foods in front of me that I loved. She stocked the refrigerator with tempting options. She sabotaged my healthy lifestyle without knowing it. Eventually, when she got on board, Julie not only began appreciating the healthy foods that I was slowly beginning to appreciate myself, but she lost 40 pounds herself. Having my wife on the same page was and is still invaluable.

FAST FOOD NATION

I list this last, but not because I underestimate the damaging effects of fast food, not even for a second. In my opinion, the fast food industry has had a hand in making America what it is today: 65 percent overweight and a place where you can make millions if you market your product creatively. In fairness, their product and movie tie-ins are well done, but too well done if pediatric obesity is at 31 percent. As I began to study nutrition and what the human body actually needed, I became mystified by the popularity of fast food. Entire generations of Americans have grown up thinking that oversized burgers with Grade F meat and deep fried potatoes are normal foods to consume daily. I learned that super-sizing was actually a marketing campaign put into play in the 1970s. It only became worse with the kids who grew up in the 80s and the kids who were born in the 90s. I have no doubt about the negative effect of fast food on me. I was the undisputed drive-thru king of the 1980s and 90s. If only I'd known then just how overdosed those foods were with calories, carbohydrates, sodium and cholesterol. One could almost assume the fast food restaurants were on a mission to make this country's kids overweight and unhealthy.

Not all that long ago I sat in a Jacuzzi at a resort in Cape Cod with my wife Julie. Below us was a massive wave pool with a slide, and seven, eight, and nine-year-old kids were lining up in droves to go on the slide. "There it is," I said to Julie.

"What?" she asked.

"There's the 31% pediatric obesity statistic lined up right in front of us," I pointed out. Indeed, every third kid in line was a "Little Gary." Problem is, "Little Gary" didn't look like that at their young age. In photos I was actually skin and bones until I was eleven. If the current generation of kids is severely overweight now, it can only get worse from here. That's my mission.

CLOSE ENCOUNTERS OF THE THERAPY KIND

As the months of my recovery from food addiction stretched on, something very troubling began happening in my life. Chronic stress and anxiety became a real problem, to the point that sleep itself, for the first time in my existence, became scarce. "They're torturing Al Qa'ida prisoners with more sleep than I'm getting these days," I quipped to my wife. Now burnout was a reality in my business, and with Harmon-Marino I'd been producing acts and creating videos, scripts and live shows for the better part of a decade. Still, it made no sense to me that at a time in my life when I was physically in better shape than I had been in years, mentally I was bottoming out. "Shouldn't the physical part carry over and give the mental part a boost?" I asked Melinda. The wealth of experience that she was, Melinda's theory on the scenario made perfect sense.

"You've turned off a major valve in your life, Gary," she said. "You used to deal with anxiety in your life by eating. That valve has been turned off for a good amount of time, and your anxiety now has nowhere else to go. No quick fix. In many ways, your mind is freaking out for a way to deal with the stress. It's perfectly normal to expect this."

It certainly made sense to me that by turning off the food pipeline I had created an anxious situation for myself. Melinda's consensus presented an interesting challenge. What do I do for a quick fix for anxiety if popping a Klondike bar is no longer an option?

Through the early phases of my recovery in 2000 and 2001, both Ruth and Melinda emphasized the importance of finding things in life, other than food, that gave me pleasure. We're talking neurological programming here, folks. The psychology of it is plain and simple: replace something in life that makes you feel good for something else that's actually good for you.

Easier said than done, right? Well, consider this. Once you've developed some habits outside the realm of junk food and alcohol, it not only can be productive, but also pretty darn therapeutic. In my case, the team had me make a list of things that made me happy in the sense that they gave me the same pleasure and satisfaction that food did. So let's jump on the therapy train and have a peek.

MONEY THERAPY

This one was a no-brainer. We're a capitalistic society, and most of us, therefore, love making money. By funneling some of the time and energy I'd normally put towards eating and cooking into my business projects, I not only did better financially, but I managed to de-emphasize the importance of food in my life. A big day at the office, such as finishing a project early or bringing in a new piece of business, feels good, and feeling good is what it's all about.

WRITING THERAPY

When I was growing up, I always loved creative writing, but by the time I was an adult, bad checks and apology letters were pretty much the only things I was writing. When Ruth and Melinda suggested I make my list, writing became an ambition again—one that was completely therapeutic and one that I could actually make money with right away. At Harmon-Marino Entertainment I had always paid comedians or writers to produce scripts or treatments whenever we had a live show to customize or a comedy video to produce. I usually paid writers, depending on the project, a fee of anywhere between $500 to $2,000. So in 2000 I made the decision, time consuming as it was, to begin handling the creative writing duties myself, thus pocketing the writing fees. And guess what? I not only discovered that I was good at it, but that it was a labor of love no different than laboring over a rack and a half of BBQ ribs. Quite a revelation!

When writing finally became a central part of my everyday life, it helped calm the food addiction. Beyond work projects, I penned letters to friends, documented my mother's passing for her grandchildren (so they wouldn't fear death as they got older) and began writing this manuscript. When the manuscript was 80 percent complete, I showed it to a select group of folks whom I knew would be objective. Most commented on the abundance of chapters in the book. My response was always the same. "Every chapter you see is therapy. It was written whenever I wanted to eat. Obviously, I wanted to eat a lot!" My advice is to write that blockbuster movie, innovative business plan, or stage theater show that's been orbiting your brain forever. It's all good energy, and even better, a distraction from food.

RETAIL THERAPY

Ladies, nothing feels better than shopping, right? Guys, let's face it, we do it too. Buying stuff on a rainy Sunday—purchasing things we want, but don't really need—the CD box set, the DVD player with surround sound, the tabloid magazine of questionable character. We all do it, and you know what? It's all good, too. A new automobile? Why, I'd love one! As long as you're not leveraging yourself to the hilt with credit cards (a financial crunch will send you running for the snack foods), treat yourself with a little retail therapy. It's fat-free, calorie-free and guilt-free food for the soul. That being said, don't put yourself into debt to avoid eating and then send me your credit card bills. We all know the saying, "Everything in moderation." Well, it applies to spending your hard earned money too!

FIX IT, BUILD IT, CLEAN IT or ORGANIZE IT THERAPY

Hey, we all know this one. Walking into a neat house after cleaning it, fixing that closet door that's hanging off its hinges, or building that shelving unit that's been in its box since Christmas—it's all good. So go ahead and wash that car, organize those kitchen cabinets, and build that gas grill. It's all therapeutic, productive, and most importantly the activity that takes your mind off eating.

PSYCHOLOGICAL THERAPY

Otherwise known as "real therapy" or "seeing a shrink." This one always has been and always will be a tough sell. It seems that no matter how old people get, they still can't get past the "You actually think I need to talk to someone?" stigma of therapy. Well, I'm here to tell you folks that we all need it, and it is the best kind of therapy there is. Telling a professional what is troubling you is empowering, liberating, and downright educational. A good therapist like Ruth will pull your feet down to earth when you complain too much, and lighten your load by helping to decipher the real problems in your life. Therapy not only distracts you from food, but also helps you to dissect your food issues in a way you may have never thought possible.

BLATANT THERAPY

And then, of course, there are the obvious ones: sex, tropical vacations, full body massages, sex, etc.

Whatever your personal interests, pursue them instead of your food interests. Like everything else, these will take time to develop. But in my opinion, finding non-food pursuits that give you the same degree of pleasure as eating is one of the most important things overweight people can do for themselves.

THE MILLION CALORIE
MARCH PROJECT

"Concern is brewing among anti-smoking advocates that their biggest private funding source for public health efforts, The Robert Wood Johnson Foundation, is bored with nicotine addiction and shifting its focus to fast food consumption."

—*U.S. News & World Report*

Around a year and a half into my addiction recovery I began thinking about how I could take all that I had learned about losing weight and give it to others. The few people in my life who have been lucky enough to beat their addictions and fix themselves always seem to move on, which to me is tragic. What is the sense of going through a life of food addiction if people can't turn a negative into a positive and help other people afflicted by the problem?

On the way down from 397 pounds, something strange began to happen around me. Family and friends who once gave me pep talks about losing weight had begun losing the battle of the bulge themselves. We've all heard of the "Freshman 15"—the fifteen pounds people normally put on during their college years. I began seeing something along the lines of the "Thirties 30" or the "Forties 45." It sure was unusual seeing people who had long lobbied, at times looking down their noses at me, for me to lose weight getting caught up in their own food issues and asking to join me for some of my walks. "How did you do it all these years?" was one humbled question. "What did it take to finally get back on track?" was another.

It was an odd twist. I figured for years I'd been inspiring these people to *stay* in shape. One look at me would put the fear of God in them to keep exercising and staying healthy. Now I was actually inspiring these same people to *get* in shape. Talk about role reversals! I deeply wanted to help these people. I no more wanted to see them go through the pain of this addiction than I wanted to go through it again myself. As with the kid on the airplane on the way home from Maui, I knew what they were in for, and I wished that pain upon no one. Ironically, when I tried to advise folks to do what I had done in hiring a support team and learning about nutrition and exercise, they usually sounded like I did 20 years ago. Some would be stubborn. "Naaaaa, I don't need to do that. Come Monday here's what I'll try…" Or they would get downright angry even talking about it. It was so strange to be on the other side of these conversations. I realized that mentally I was miles ahead of these folks, but I had no way of pushing their inner buttons. That had to come from them. Inspiration seemed to be one thing I could provide, and I had some ideas on how I could give it. In my heart I felt that if I could light the fire under even one person I could come to terms with the years I'd spent hopelessly stuck in self-destruct mode, addicted to the drug known as food.

Men in particular seem in need of inspiration. The weight loss industry has been around for 50 years or better, yet it all seems to be geared towards women and their eating disorders. For whatever reason, overweight guys are simply not out buying books, videos or joining weight loss programs. Not that anything is geared towards the average overweight guy with a food addiction, but think about it. Millions of American men are dealing with weight problems, and still the bulk of the business is geared towards the other gender. This has always been an interesting phenomenon to me. Even from my early days at places like Weight Watchers, the guys were always pretty scarce. Somehow it has become un-masculine for males to seek any sort of help. Then again, you can never actually picture a big dude in his robe on Christmas morning opening gifts and saying, "Thanks for the DVD player and the Richard Simmons 'Sweating To The Oldies' disc. I love them both!"

I mulled over the possible ideas for entire days at a time. Make a self-help video? Easy enough, owning my own production company, but at this point I was hardly a weight loss guru. Start a Jenny Craig like walk-in clinic? Naaa. You all know by now how well that approach worked for me. Maybe I'd start…

"The All new Weight Loss Channel"

Twenty-four hours a day of shows to watch whenever you are hungry. Tonight at 5:00, double episodes of ER, followed by the first 30 minutes of "Saving Private

Ryan"! Then immediately following, it's a triple feature beginning with "Mask" at 7:00, "Alive" at 8:30, wrapping up with "Schindler's List" at 10:00!

And for you late night eaters, don't forget that our open-heart surgery programming begins at midnight!

"The Weight Loss Channel" probably could have worked for people, but I began to focus on some ideas that were a little more practical.

One day, while mulling over several possibilities with my Uncle Dave in his office, we came up with an idea for a unique, cross-country weight loss walk. The country had already experienced walks for breast cancer, AIDS and MS, but nobody appeared to be doing one for obesity. The weight loss walk would cover over 1200 miles, raise awareness, and inspire a huge percentage of people who had given up hope on ever achieving their health goals to succeed. The walk would also raise funds for a foundation I would start to help battle obesity. "Highway to Health" was one name we tossed around. "Million Calorie March" was another. I liked the latter. It was a humorous name, but appropriate for a serious cause as well. The walk, which would be the first of its kind, would begin in Jacksonville, FL and end in Boston, MA near the site of the famous Boston Marathon finish line. The concept was as easy as this. If, as a lifelong overweight food addict, I could complete a daunting physical challenge such as a Million Calorie March right up the eastern seaboard, then perhaps it would inspire people right in their own hometowns to find their own Million Calorie Marches. I wouldn't necessarily suggest that ordinary folks drop everything and walk across the country like me, but hopefully I would inspire them to dig down deep and develop their own unique approaches to getting healthy. I figured that with 61 percent of the country struggling with weight problems, the epidemic was out of control. One look at the newspaper headlines and it was clear that the time was right for a unique awareness campaign. Most health experts were calling for a massive public relations effort (similar to the anti-tobacco campaign) to turn the obesity epidemic around, and I decided I would champion their cause.

My uncle and I strategized that corporate sponsorship, pledge money and private donations could help fund the costs of "The March." We plotted a "measles map" with stops along the way at state capitols, health forums, wellness centers such as ViQuest in North Carolina, and institutions such as the Duke University Weight Loss Center. Although I would be the only one completing the entire 1200 mile walk, I hoped that I'd be joined by many people along the way;

namely, anyone who believed in the cause or wanted to walk off a few pounds. I began educating myself on pediatric obesity and searching for ways in which the foundation might be able to help. In July I traveled to Camp Kingsmont, a weight loss camp for kids in the Berkshire Mountains of Massachusetts. Kingsmont had been receiving national media coverage on TV shows such as "Good Morning America" and magazines such as *People*. The owners of the camp graciously invited me to observe the daily happenings and I was immediately impressed. The camp embraced a successful mix of de-emphasizing food without denying it. Additionally, they operated with the mindset that if children were encouraged to find an exercise they loved, they would stick with it for life. Whether it was tennis, soccer, baseball, racquetball or jogging, the activity would be a crucial part of their future health goals as they become adults. Toward the end of my visit, I observed an interesting meeting between "Shape Down" (the in-house weight counselors) and a handful of parents. At the private outside gathering, concerned moms and dads were educated on how to properly handle their kids' mounting weight problems. They were taught that the wrong approach would only exacerbate the problem and send their kids running for more food. The meeting was extremely thought-provoking and informative, and yet very low key. One concerned mother asked, "How do I deal with my other kids who are not overweight but feel punished if I don't buy foods such as ice cream and chips?"

"What is the best way to handle second helpings at the dinner table?" asked another.

One father asked the million-dollar question. "My kid seems to know he's coming here to lose weight every summer, so he doesn't even try to eat healthy and exercise during the school year. How should I handle this?"

Parents were learning how to handle their kids' food issues. Fascinating concept. The campers came from cities and towns up and down the East Coast and the management of Kingsmont felt strongly that their campers would be interested in joining me along the walk route. I pledged to use some of the money raised by the walk to fund tuitions and educational tools for the camp. As I drove home through the gorgeous green hills of the Berkshires, my mind raced with ideas about educational tapes and DVDs our foundation could produce for parents and kids alike, all funded by the Million Calorie March (MCM) project.

Just as Harmon-Marino had begun to take on a life of its own quite a few years earlier, the cross-country walk seemed to be headed on the same course. The people working on the project with me were excited. Public relations contacts and driver possibilities were dropping in and out of my office almost weekly. We designed proposals for corporate sponsorship and retained a lawyer to cover the legal issues. My assistant began researching potential companies who could donate startup money, clothing, supplies and food, as well as the mobile home. Everybody around me chimed in with advice and contacts. I hired some of my freelance cameramen to help shoot background video, which would not only serve as a sponsorship video but could be used in a documentary film we hoped to make about the project. Matty Blake, one of my management clients, approached me to direct the initial sponsorship video. Matty had a unique understanding and compassion for addicts following his own family's struggle with alcohol. I had noticed his flair for directing a year earlier when I hired him to write and act in a series of comedy videos for the Stop & Shop Corporation. The two of us were friends from that day back in '97 when we commenced working together. I could not think of a better person to direct the Million Calorie March video. Matt had a passion for what I was trying to do, and he did a sensational job.

By late summer 2001, the MCM project was accelerating at a phenomenal rate and a good portion of my work days were being spent on the walk. I hired consultants like Stephen Warshaw and David McGillivray. Stephen owned a successful company named Moving Experiences, which not only managed nationwide events such as the G.E. Women's Health Tour, but coordinated sponsorships as well. At our meetings, I was fascinated by Steve's creativity and tie-in ideas. He taught me how to make the event work for the sponsors first and our cause second. I was like a sponge around Steven Warshaw. Having worked in the sponsorship arena with some impressive Fortune 500 companies, he was truly amazing.

David McGillivray's accomplishments were impressive as well. In 1978 he completed the first-ever run from Medford, Oregon to Medford, Massachusetts, all to benefit The Jimmy Fund. At the finish line, a chubby 13-year-old (you guessed it, me!) patted Dave on the back and congratulated him on his run. By the time I'd sought Dave out for my project, he had completed a Florida-to-Boston run of his own, as well as built a busy sports marketing company called DMSE, Inc. Dave McGillivray believed that the project could fly and was gracious in offering pro bono advice. It would not be easy, but by now I realized that nothing great in life ever is.

Vinnie Sestito, my longtime friend and client, spent many endless nights with me, designing the Million Calorie March marketing pieces. One of the pieces was a shot of me walking into the sunset on a long winding road. The caption at the top read "Sometimes Inspiration Can Come From The Most Unlikely People." How true that statement was! A 300-pound man turning the eastern seaboard into his own personal treadmill doesn't happen every day. And did I ever, throughout any of this, question my own sanity? You can count on it.

Despite everything, the thought of putting together a walk of this type excited me. Not only would I come home a very different person, but I figured I could light a spark which could ignite others affected by the disease.

By the fall of 2001, the project was beginning to grow some legs and I was determined to see it succeed. If there was a selfish reason for undertaking the project, I guess it was simply that I knew being involved in the obesity issue would help keep me focused on my personal health for the long term. My reasons for doing it, however, were centered around inspiring as many people as I possibly could. Getting the project off the ground did not come cheap. By September I'd already invested a good deal of my own money. On a positive note, however, I'd begun to garner serious interest from a handful of national companies to sponsor the cross-country walk.

We researched companies whose products were a good match. Energy bars, water companies, footwear giants, pedometer makers, retailers of health related products, etc. Even secondary needs were targets: sun screen companies, clothing makers, tires for the mobile home, laptop computers to update the web site. Chafing, anyone? How about our friends over at "Bond's Gold Powder"? The list of potential sponsors for the project continued to grow, and when I was lucky enough to get the decision makers on the line, the phone calls usually went like this.

ME: "Hello, Mr. So & so. I'm walking from Florida to Boston next year to…"

POTENTIAL SPONSOR: "You know you can take a bus for that…"

These conversations, however, always ended with people agreeing to at least take a look at my event. That said, I also kept a realistic outlook on my chances of pulling off an event like the Million Calorie March. Never for a minute did I think the MCM would be easy, from a business perspective. Even with all of the people and energy around the project, there was a cautious tone as I went about my work. Privately, I asked the people around me, as well as my family, to keep "low key" about the event until I was certain it had financial backing and was feasible. I had no illusions. Sponsorship had always been a long shot. Unfortunately, as we all know, family can sometimes get over-excited and forget certain requests, such as keeping something "low key." I knew I was in trouble when I walked into my brother's restaurant one night with a client and received a standing ovation. *Uh oh,* I remember thinking. *I better actually pull this one off.* Another time a friend of my dad asked Julie if she was the daughter-in-law "married to the million-dollar guy." Just when I figured the misadventures had stopped, my life was like a bad sitcom again. There I would be, walking out of the supermarket and so and so' s brother-in-law hits me with "Ayyyyyy! When are you leaving for your Million Mile Walk?" People I barely knew would walk up to me at weddings and say things like "I hear you're going on a long trek." So much for "low key." Nothing like your own family upping the ante when you're already feeling the pressure, right? I had to smile. Their hearts were in the right place and they were excited about what I was planning. Despite all the energy around the project, my instincts for some reason told me the Million Calorie March would not be on the fast track.

On the morning of September 11, 2001, I was driving along sunny Memorial Drive in Cambridge with one of my longtime cameramen. We were en-route to the famous Bull & Finch Pub in downtown Boston for an 8:45 a.m. meeting. The Bull & Finch had been the inspiration for the long running "Cheers" sitcom on NBC, and I'd been in talks with them to produce a pair of colorful training videos for their employees. I was not surprised to see tourists and sight-seeing crowds both outside and inside of the pub when we arrived, yet there was a distinct heaviness in the air as we made our way through the crowd towards the restaurant where we were meeting with the managers. People everywhere seemed to be stopped in their tracks, watching the TV monitors which normally ran "Cheers" re-runs.

As we quietly squeezed through the crowds and followed our clients to a table in the corner of the restaurant, I caught a quick glimpse of what was on the television monitor. Either "Cheers" had run out of plots and made an episode about a horrific fire in New York City, or the World Trade Center Towers were on fire. It was 9:00 a.m. Like the folks glued to the monitors, my head was in shock and my heart was sinking. The gravity of the situation had not completely hit me yet. Once we arrived at the table and sat down, it was clear that nobody was really interested in talking business. We were all watching the scenes unfold on the monitors, and everybody at the table was glued. The project had been dragging on for months at that point, so I made a half-hearted attempt to present my ideas for the videos. "I've got two on-camera talents in mind to host the videos and I think both would do a great…" *BOOM!* Split screen. Bryant Gumbel is talking about a terrorist hit on New York and the Pentagon being on fire in Washington. "The meeting's over," said my client as he stood up and motioned to his people to follow him back upstairs to the executive suites. My cameraman and I gathered up our stuff and joined the crowd over by the monitors.

Tower One fell. The world as we knew it was changing forever. I watched with every other American as reporters described the brutal airplane hijackings of flights originating from Boston's Logan Airport, just a mile or so from where we stood. Tower Two collapsed. We headed for a quick walk in the Boston Public Gardens across the street to try to shake off the sick feelings we had. As we did, we looked up at the Prudential and John Hancock Towers in the Boston skyline. The morning sun was out and the gardens around us were green and healthy. A warm, gentle breeze was blowing. It was a beautiful day, and yet we could not take our eyes off those tall buildings.

As the week of September 11th dragged on, my aggressive plans for a cross-country walk to raise awareness for obesity began to seem pretty trivial compared to what was going on in the world. My healthy eating continued, but like everyone else, I sat glued to the television screen for days, waiting to see how the country would rise up.

It had become apparent that the attacks had not only impacted the nation's psyche, but the already weakened economy. Jobs were being eliminated, sponsorship budgets were being slashed everywhere, and if not completely wiped out, sponsors were redirecting their dollars towards more patriotic efforts to rally the country after the brutal attacks. At Harmon-Marino, cancellations had brought business to a complete standstill for the first time in a decade. At that point, most of the folks working with me on the Million Calorie March seemed to say the same thing: put the project on hiatus until the country is ready to concentrate on issues other than the war on terror. I couldn't agree more. Who cared about a big guy walking down the highway to inspire folks to lose weight when people were running around New York City with anti-Anthrax masks strapped to their faces?

By late fall, with the country still on a heightened state of alert, the war on terror dragging on and the economy getting worse by the day, the inaction was beginning to get to me. My own weight loss goals were beginning to slip, and I began to realize just how therapeutic all that work on the MCM had been for me. It had, in fact, kept my motivation going strong. Now everything seemed to be at a standstill.

Making the MCM sponsorship video was instrumental in helping me face myself and my disease. Putting my struggle out there in a very public way had strengthened my resolve and I began searching for something that would be equally as therapeutic until it was time for the MCM project to come alive again. One day I began to read some of my weight loss journals from the previous year. From day one, Melinda had asked me to keep track of not only what I ate, but also what I was feeling at the time. Ruth had requested a similar record, this one more geared toward the psychology of my eating at any given time. Early on, Julie had designed a daily journal on the desktop for me to keep track of everything. Around mid-November I began to notice that my journals, if punched up, could be not only educational, but at times pretty amusing reading as well, especially for those involved in the struggle with addiction recovery. I decided to document my daily experiences (normal, abnormal, on the wagon, off the wagon, etc.) and create a manuscript. What happened was more than therapeutic. It was the equivalent of producing a weight loss video everyday. It became a permanent part of my day and helped me to further dissect my disorder. Through the writing process, I truly began to understand the psychology of my food addiction, where I had been in my life, and how the toxic environment had derailed my health goals during all those years. Now throughout my life, folks had been giving me diet and self-help books to read, hoping they'd help me to see the light. The truth is the books all sounded the same and never quite held my attention. I decided that with mine, I would incorporate equal parts of humor and heartache and create a manuscript that I would have read even in my worst stages of denial. I also set out to reach the "big guys" out there who might have felt alienated by the weight loss industry's multi-year, women-only marketing strategies. It was always an eyebrow raiser to me. Magazines, products, infomercials, you name it, they were all geared towards the female gender. It was no secret that it was women who were buying the products and signing up for the programs, but I felt if I could reach both genders, it would be a significant breakthrough. The reality was that plenty of males were struggling as well. Writing my sometimes painfully entertaining weight battle memoirs ultimately gave me the strength and resolve to pursue my mission, in spite of being derailed by the events surrounding 9/11. With the cross-country walk on indefinite hiatus, I began to put into play the other parts of my project—the parts that I knew I could make happen even without support from corporate sponsors.

I began designing the foundation, which eventually became Generation Excel, to develop and create action programs aimed at educating overweight children and their parents. Pop culture, as well as the media, had been referring to the overweight youth of the 1990s and 2000s as Generation XL (extra large). Julie came up with the idea to put a positive spin on it and change it to "Excel." I envisioned an interactive website, with the experts who had helped me dispensing helpful advice online: "Ask The Nutritionist" pages; "Ask the Therapist"; "Ask the Fitness Trainer." The foundation could also fund gym memberships for kids and obesity clinics along the lines of the Dr. Lee Kaplan's center at Massachusetts General Hospital. Since many schools had cut gym and physical fitness programs, I figured we could pay for part-time instructors to return those very important classes to the schools. My old friend Boston City Councilor John Tobin had been working on an initiative to remove vending machines from the schools. I approached John to partner with me on the gym teachers for schools idea as a pilot program, and he immediately agreed. Maybe we could even assist in lobbying efforts aimed at creating government action programs that could bring about real change. I wrote a treatment for an educational and instructional DVD for parents of overweight kids titled, what else? "Waisted Youth." Once a year perhaps the foundation could even select one American in need of help and take them on a "Mini-Million Calorie March" to get them healthy. Ideas? I had a million of them as far as making a difference, but non-profit foundations are a dime a dozen. I decided that if I was going to design one, it would be a foundation that would truly impact this problem. It might not happen overnight, but future generations could be saved from being "waisted."

Of course, as I spent long nights designing the foundation and writing about my experiences, I had to laugh about how things had changed. During all those early years I was so unapproachable on the subject of weight. I was never in denial about it, just inapproachable. Now I couldn't talk about the subject enough. A healing had begun, the likes of which even my partners and friends involved in the Million Calorie March project could not have foreseen.

One day soon, I'll get back to the 1200-mile cross-country walk. I may be 185 pounds by that time and it may be called the Million Calorie Run, but I'll get back to it. Anyone who knows me knows that determination and resolve have always been some of my strongest attributes. One way or another, I'll head out on that highway to join the fight against obesity, and at the same time do some personal cleansing of my own. I'll do it because it touched a lot of people during its planning stages. The idea of the MCM challenge walk gave people hope. In America, we are in dire need of help to turn the obesity crisis around. We need grassroots support as well as help from big corporations and politicians. The event may be without all the hype and fanfare, but sooner or later the Million Calorie March will happen. And when it does, I'll see you on the road.

50 THE HARD WAY

By Thanksgiving of 2001, I had dropped fifty pounds—the hard way. No quick fixes, no compliments or fanfare (frankly it wasn't all that noticeable physically), and no new scientific breakthroughs. Just me and my Walkman, exercising every-day that I could and literally spending hundreds of hours with my weight loss dream team, dissecting my every habit and learning facts about the world of health that I had long been ignoring.

For example, the amount of time it takes for the average adult to burn one McDonald's super-sized meal? How about 6 hours. The best way to kick-start your metabolism? Eat six or seven small meals throughout the day versus the usual three. This information had always been there, I just needed to want to learn it. There were no regrets about my earlier ignorance nor repenting for the years I had spent as a hopeless food addict, just an older Gary with a new attitude and a realistic approach to getting healthy. I began noticing and studying the people in my life who were both healthy and in great shape. I liked their energy and was attracted to the glow that emanated from them, the way they were able to do just about anything physically and still seem young, and the way they carried themselves. I wanted into that club. The little kid in me wanted to be part of that clubhouse. There was a deep desire to succeed this time. I knew the desire would be there even if I fell off my path. There would always be days when I would fall back into my old ways, but I had a powerful new confidence that I could get myself back on track before my pursuit of food developed into a self-destructive lifestyle again. I had already lived that lifestyle, and there was no future in it. I wanted to walk, even when I knew I had just eaten something way off of my health regimen. There was nothing I could do about the years I had spent as an overweight guy. At this point I have spent most of my teens, twenties and half of my thirties looking like Elvis on his last tour in the 1970s. I can't get those years back, but I relish the idea of hitting forty looking and feeling better than I ever did in my twenties and thirties. That would be a measurable degree of payback, and I would also escape the unavoidable long-term effects of obesity. Heck, I might even *live* to be forty! I once asked Melinda if I should learn to hate and resent food for what it had done to my life. She answered, "No, you shouldn't hate food, because that's not realistic. Food is good and it will always be there. You should hate what your approach to food has done to your life." I understood what she was talking about. Life was not my personal all-you-can-eat buffet, and the "All or Nothing" syndrome was now beginning to seem stupid to me. At 348 pounds, a 50-pound obstacle had been removed and my clothes were now hanging off me. If only I had a nickel for every time I had walked in with groceries, only to have my pants hanging down around my knees, I'd be a rich man. But whether or not I was rich, my face and body surely looked leaner. Well, perhaps "leaner" is the wrong word. I looked less bloated. Not quite as puffy. I felt much better, had more energy and was able to think more clearly now. Life's daily challenges were simply not as daunting.

The change was so slow that you could not exactly feel it overnight. It was not instant. I had to constantly recall what I felt like before the weight loss in order to observe the change. It was a process of slowly getting better each day. If we could all be at our goal weight for even one day to experience what that would feel like, we would all be itching to get there. Unfortunately, weight loss is not like that. It is a process of very slowly feeling better each day. The old me would have been discouraged that for all my efforts I was still over 300 pounds. The old me would have dive-bombed off of the health regimen because it was "hopeless, painfully slow, and just not in the cards this year." But that inner button had been pushed and my resolve was stronger than ever. I also had given up alcohol for good. For years, drinking had simply been the garnish on my plateful of self-destruction. If you've been reading this, you know I drank my share of beers, but throughout the years I never felt addicted to it. Hey, I already had my addiction. How many does a guy need? The truth is, the taste never really appealed to me, and the bloat was no fun either. Who could possibly miss the bloat factor from drinking alcohol? I just didn't need it. "You're not drinking tonight?" friends would occasionally ask me.

"Hey, I feel like hell as it is with all this weight on, I don't need help," I'd quip. Giving up booze was the easiest part of the weight loss experience for me. By the age of 25 I had slowly begun to lose any desire to do it. Unless I was spending the weekend with my in-laws, of course. But that's a story for another book.

The actual weight loss was not the significant change I experienced throughout the process. Rather, it was the unyielding resolve that I had achieved over a sustained period of time. Never in my life had I maintained the eye of the tiger for that amount of time while simultaneously learning as much as I could about eating healthy and exercising. Melinda and Ruth constantly reminded me that the next 50 pounds would bring more of the results I wanted. To most thin people, 298 pounds would not be reason to celebrate, but to me it represented the weight I was while in college, and it called for a complete wardrobe change. I also knew that I would have even more energy and a sharper mental focus. And finally, it would put me within striking distance of my next goal: 250 pounds, a weight at which I could vividly remember being comfortable and happy. Bring it on.

GIRTH ANNOUNCEMENTS:
Staying Away From the Numbers

There are a few guilty pleasures in life, like listening to early Madonna, watching the Yankees get stomped by the Red Sox, or witnessing Saddam being pulled out of a spider hole. Another is being able to talk publicly about your recent weight loss. It's like hitting the lottery. You're on top of your game. And boy, do folks love talking to a guy who's on top of his weight game. Maybe it's because they all know how hard it really is to overcome a serious obstacle like food addiction, or maybe it's because they told you that you needed to lose weight years ago. (You just apparently didn't listen!) Who knows? It's an interesting phenomenon. You can be a convicted criminal in America, but if you're losing weight successfully, we love ya! You look great!

As early as 13, I was jumping on scales and publicly reporting my weight loss to people. They always seemed to want to know. "Half a pound! Beautiful!" I'd rejoice. "Anybody up for a deep dish pizza?" As long as I'd lost something, you know? You can be almost anywhere in America today and you'll hear people asking, "How much are you down?" We love it. It's like a stock market where everybody comes out on top. Music to our ears. The USA is the greatest country to live in, but we're obsessed with the polar opposites these days—namely eating lots of food and losing lots of weight.

I love America, but why is it we can't accept that Mama Cass—the super-sized singer from "The Mamas & The Papas"—died from heart failure stemming from excess in all areas? Why will we only accept the idea that due to her excessive *eating*, she choked on a massive sandwich in her hotel room? By the same token, there are probably people in Memphis touring Graceland right at this moment who think Elvis Presley, in his signature ballad "Love Me Tender," was singing about chicken tenders. As a society, we are simply obsessed with eating food and losing weight: two things that essentially cancel each other out.

By my 30s I had pretty much decided it was better to stay away from talking about my weight loss with people in actual pounds. Girth announcements are fun at first, but eventually they become a double-edged sword. Let me give you an example. Someone notices you've been losing weight. First they'll begin with a compliment: "You look great, what a difference!" Then they'll ask (and they *always* ask), "How much have you lost, anyway?" You'll respond 10, 20, 50, 80 pounds, or whatever it is. Their next comment will typically be something like, "That much? You had that much to lose? Well, what did you let yourself get up to anyway?" Do you see what just happened? We just went from a compliment to an insult in no time at all. Now you're standing there, actually embarrassed for ever letting yourself go in the first place. It's like you plea-bargained down from first-degree compliment to second-degree involuntary insult! What happened? You gave the numbers, and most people—especially those who have never been through it—can't fathom the notion that you ever gained it or lost it.

I've seen this scenario unfold many times with my own weight, as well as with others, and it's the same every time. Starts with a compliment, ends with an insult.

Here's another one. Someone comments that you look as if you've slimmed down. You respond by thanking them and informing them of the weight loss in actual pounds. "Yeah, I'm down about a hundred right now," you say.

Then they backslap you with a line like "Oh yeah, I can see it in your face, it's really slimmed down." Now you're just plain insulted. *My face? You think I look like I lost 100 pounds off my head? You don't see the weight loss anywhere else on my body?* Again, compliment to an insult, because you invoked the numbers, completely unsolicited.

Now most people do not intend to be negative or hurtful, but in reality, such comments can be detrimental to your cause. They can weaken your resolve and deflate you emotionally. For all you emotional eaters out there, it's the stuff that leads to Post-Traumatic Stretch Disorder. We get emotional because we've been insulted, so we make a dash for our friends, Ben & Jerry.

Your weight loss is a personal health situation. You're not under obligation to release facts and figures to anyone who notices your physical appearance. Take their compliments about looking better and move on. Don't get into the numbers game with friends, family, or anybody else. If you do, they'll want to know exactly how much you've lost since the last girth announcement, like you're some kind of walking Jerry Lewis Telethon, announcing figures as they come in. Or you're a question on The Family Feud. "Most Americans believe that you personally need to lose more weight. Survey says…" But realistically, there is another reason to stay away from the numbers. You shouldn't be overly obsessed with what you weigh and how much you've lost. You're losing inches, toning your body, gaining muscle and changing mentally. You are also learning a process that just may be the most important thing you learn in your life: how to kick the addiction, achieve life balance and, ultimately, find happiness.

On Thanksgiving a couple of years ago, my sister gave me a hug when I walked in the door and told me I looked awesome, in front of a room full of people. Even though I steered clear of talking numbers, I was initially embarrassed. There was just something ridiculous about weighing 350 pounds and having someone actually tell me I looked awesome, but I knew where she was coming from. She didn't need to know the numbers. It wasn't even about that. No girth announcements were needed. I was a guy who was finally on his way. And *that* was awesome!

RELAPSE:
STOPPING THE MADNESS

It was a warm Saturday in November, 2001. Julie and I were having company over for dinner. "See some old friends, good for the soul," as Bob Seger once so nicely put it. We hit the local meat market to buy marinated steak tips for our dinner guests. Already I was in a perverse place for someone like me. This particular place made steak tips so good people actually ate them straight off the grill. The tips looked so good that I stood in line, thanking God that they were sold raw. When we hit the register I reached for my wallet to pay. Almost on cue a woman walked over and set a huge tray of BBQ cheesesteak calzones right on the register. Did I mention that these slices of calzone are hot out of the oven and 75 cents per slice? *Oh wow, my old friends. You had me at "hello."* I turned and looked at Julie. It's not even a negotiable issue. *I've got to have one. I'm in the calzone zone. $1,000 bucks a slice? No problem. Money's no object. So long, eye of the tiger, hello eye of the addict!* I bought us each a slice. I needed a partner in crime, you know. Suddenly it was the old me again, sitting in my car, eating that slice right out of the oven. If you love food, you know exactly what I'm talking about. No regrets. I devoured the slice with no guilt whatsoever. I had my fix. A justifiable loss of control.

Our next stop was the supermarket to pick up some additional groceries for our dinner party. I was being good now. I picked up fruit for the coming week. Pineapple cottage cheese for breakfast and a pound of turkey breast for sandwiches during the week. Spring water for the office. Pretty good, right? I was back on track. As I headed past the dairy section to get eggs, I caught a package out of the corner of my eye. I rolled the carriage back to take a closer look and could not believe what I was seeing: Kraft Foods, the makers of fine cheese products everywhere, had done it. They'd really gone and done it. They'd come out with a raspberry cheesecake bar, chilled, wrapped and ready to eat. 6 to a box. It's all over. I looked at Julie and fondled the box as if it contained gold bars. Once again, I was over the top. *The nerve of these people to come out with such a good product,* I thought. *Now I may end up doing something I'll regret in the morning.* Cheesecake should be reserved for special occasions, only to be eaten in a cake form, not a readily available candy bar version, right? And this version was auto-friendly, much like the calzone. Now I know I've said I was never much of a sweets guy, but heck, I'll drive to a New York City deli for the right slice of cheesecake, and these people offer this product right in the local dairy section.

For the second time in less than an hour, I looked at Julie and threw it in the carriage. It would have come to blows if she'd tried to stop me. Julie knew better than to get between me and my addiction. I was off. The old Gary was back. One show only, folks. He's baaack.

Again we got back to the car and unloaded the groceries into the trunk. Well, most of the groceries. Those cheesecake bars were riding up front with me as far as I was concerned. Even *I* couldn't believe how focused and obsessed I was. I slid into the driver's seat and cracked that baby open. Wow, was it good! Almost orgasmic. Suddenly it was like the *Million Calorie March,* which had always been a metaphor for my journey to health, had never happened. I realized I was dangerously close to "ALL" mode again. I knew I had to stop the madness. I called my cousin Michele, who knew the "ALL" mode almost as well as I did. If this was a 12-step program, I guess you'd call her my sponsor. "You've got to help me!" I pleaded from my cell phone. Michele laughed at my story and came up with some great advice. "Eat two bars and throw the rest away," she advised. "That way you won't feel cheated for buying them, but you'll have them out of your life." Great plan. I loved it. I wanted them out of my life. I felt myself running with the wrong crowd again. I knew I'd worked too hard to go down this track. Speaking of tracks, adjacent to the supermarket parking lot were train tracks. The trains run hourly into Boston. I bolted out of the car and up the train tracks, leaving Michele on the cell phone on the dashboard. I was desperate. I ran 50 yards up the tracks until I was out of sight and then threw the box right on the track. There I was, a grown man committing a cheesecake bar massacre. Within an hour, I knew they'd all be dead. I walked back to the car victoriously. The dream had been realized and once again I was in control. A free man once more.

TOP HALF-DOZEN OBESITY FELONIES

I thought at this point I'd take a break from the "Misadventures" to remind folks just how out of whack the world has gotten with the whole weight issue. Most Americans find the subject of losing weight interesting to watch and learn about, but few, including myself, find it *entertaining*. That is, of course, unless you look at what's going on out there in the media these days; then it's the stuff David Letterman's Top Ten Lists are made of. So here goes my "Top Half Dozen Obesity Felonies" in the media. Keep in mind that these are simply my observations, and they are not the reasons I decided to get healthy. Nevertheless, they are inspirational in a funny if-this-is-what-it's-come-to sort of way.

1. Lawsuit Against Fast Food Chains

Wow, what a time to be a standup comedian in America! Back in 1998 Bill Clinton and Monica Lewinsky were God's gift to comedians. Then in 2002, just when it seemed the country was beginning to accept obesity as a true blue disease, a disgruntled group of overweight folks launched a high profile suit against fast-food chains such as McDonald's, Wendy's and Kentucky Fried Chicken, accusing these companies of serving foods that led to their obesity. Other complaints held that the chains did not clearly advertise what was in their foods. Now in sue-happy America, I've always believed that the fast food industry was ripe for some type of lawsuit, but not necessarily for obesity. How can you sue someone for the choices that you yourself made? If that's the case, perhaps I should sue Salem State College for contributing to my lack of a six-figure salary? If my home depreciates in value, maybe I can sue the real estate company? Of course not. Nor can I sue the maker of the computer I'm writing this on, which took six attempts to boot up for me this morning. The felony is not the lawsuit itself, but in my opinion it is the way the media treats the case. Indeed, once word leaked out about the suit, every comic from Jay Leno ("Word is they are forming a Million Pound March on Washington") to a little-known comic from Boston ("I think a good step toward eliminating the grievances of these insatiable carnivores would be to eliminate the drive-through window") began jumping on the frenzy of available cheap shots. Even newspapers could not resist a good old all-American cheap shot, with editorials like "This Fat Guy Doesn't Deserve a Break Today" and "Fat Chance These Plaintiffs Will Opt for Tofu Over Burgers." Eventually, the case was dismissed and fast food was spared from being labeled a "controlled substance." Just when it looked like the lawsuits would do for obesity what Johnnie "OJ Simpson" Cochran did for race relations, a silver lining appeared. In the months and weeks that followed the dismissal, the fast food industry, wary of the negative press, began rethinking their product lines and began creating healthier alternatives and branding for health. Not a bad ending after all.

2. Jared, the Subway Sandwich Boy

Having read Jared's personal story, I'm skeptical. 245 pounds lost in one year? That's healthy. Only a cup of coffee for breakfast? Talk about breaking rule number one of losing weight: eat breakfast! A sub for lunch, and then another for dinner and not much else in between? Purely ridiculous. Now for those of us struggling with eating disorders most of our lives, the concept of losing weight eating submarine sandwiches is another in a long line of laughable approaches. Adding insult to injury, of course, the other not-so-healthy chains began to see the branding value in Jared. They started their own searches for pitchmen willing to say they got to their goal weights eating cereal, fried chicken and God-knows-what-else. About the only way a campaign like this could have been more insulting is if "Blimpie" subs had come up with it. Do we really need a guy holding sliced turkey grinders up to the camera lens? Well, maybe if they're Italian cold cut…But I digress. Personally, I'd believe that you could lose weight at Subway if they had one key ingredient, that being extremely attractive individuals working behind the counter. I think most overweight people know what I'm talking about here. You walk in with every intention of ordering the largest greasy sub available, but as soon as the gorgeous manager behind the counter asks, "Can I help you?" you automatically down-grade your order to the garden salad with low-cal, fat-free, taste-free dressing. Now that's a distraction, folks. And I personally *know* it works.

3. Fat Assassin Pills

In the winter of 1998, radio commercials for this miracle weight loss product were in heavy (no pun intended, this is radio talk) rotation on fine radio stations across New England. I have two problems with this product. First, it doesn't work. Second, its name: Fat Assassin? Is this what it's come down to? All these years I've been dealing with a weight problem and apparently all I had to do was hire an assassin. Who knew?

Like all the other shameless scam products in the already flooded marketplace, this product doesn't work either. The reason some innocent consumers might be losing weight is because they are in a temporary healthy state of mind. They're walking, exercising, eating healthy and taking this product everyday to get fit. Here's a concept, people: walk, exercise and eat healthy every day. I'll guarantee you'll lose the same amount without the "Fat Assassin." That magical pill we all have been waiting for is never coming, folks, the one we pop before each meal and actually lose weight afterward. It's not coming because the only true way to lose weight is what's been around from the beginning: reducing carbohydrates and calories, and exercising.

4. Southwest Airline's "Body Profiling"

Destined to make the public relations bloopers reel someday, in the summer of 2002 this airline announced to the media that they would begin a new policy of charging overweight people for an extra seat. "Body profiling," they called it. Here's how it worked. Airline employees would inspect the passengers beforehand. If they surmised that a person would not fit into the 18-inch seat, they would pull them out of line and charge them for the cost of two seats. Thanks, folks. As if the flying experience wasn't already humiliating enough for obese people. As if airplane seats weren't already the fat man's straightjacket, let's charge more money and cause a scene while you're at it! As if asking for a seatbelt extension wasn't embarrassing enough, let's kick it up a notch. Let's have air marshals spend their time physically weighing people in the terminals. "Go ahead, Mr. Terrorist, you're all set. Excuse me, sir, we'll need to measure your butt before you board." Why not extend the policy to the pilots? If they're overweight, should we ban them from the flight as well? Seriously, airplane seats are uncomfortable for most *thin* people I know. Now here's the airline industry, fresh from a fifteen-billion-dollar federal bailout, attempting to make more money. Here's another idea for the folks at Southwest. Force overweight people to eat those subpar airline meals for six months. Heck, we'll all be able to fit!

5. Scam Diet Radio Pitchmen

Can't we as a society put a limit on the amount of weight loss product endorsements one radio personality can do? In Boston we've got several who have been doing this for years. For those of us truly battling food addiction, it's kind of insulting. One month they are all over the airwaves, talking about some new "breakthrough" product that has finally and quite easily taken off their weight. "It did it for me and it can do it for you. Just call 1-800…" The problem is, these people aren't really losing weight because of the product. If they are losing, it's because, once again, the product has them in a temporarily healthy state of mind. Eventually the ads stop running and I run into these folks buffalo-stancing a buffet somewhere around town. It's very predictable and pretty nauseating when these very same radio types turn up six months later only to promote a new "miracle weight loss product that really works this time. No diets, no exercise necessary. Just call 1-800…" Hello? Weren't you just promoting another product? Didn't you call the last product "the cure to your weight problem once and for all?" And of course these folks could care less. The deal is the weight loss company donates the product for free and the radio personality gets their own commercials on the air in heavy rotation, which is what it's all really about anyway. Some of these folks have been laboring away in obscurity most of their careers. Now they feel they can get thin and hear themselves on the radio every commercial break. Some of these people are on their fourth and fifth product endorsements, which wouldn't bother me so much if they weren't 400 and 500 pounds. Stop the insanity, or at least the vanity.

6. The "Chocolate Is Good for You" Study

Boy, haven't we come full circle in this country when chocolate—that's right, *chocolate*—is now supposed to be good for you? In a study released to the press on February 16, 2002, it was announced that chocolate now has certain medical benefits, including aiding in the prevention of blood clots, almost the same way baby aspirin does. Who knew? All this time it was healthy for me. Of course, while I'm venting here, let's add the fact that to most people struggling with their weight, chocolate is and always has been the absolute devil. Evil in a candy wrapper. Lucifer in a Count Chocula outfit. Now, after all these years of denying ourselves, it's suddenly healthy. Quick, someone do a study on blue cheese and eggnog. Boy I miss those two. But hold on a minute. Before you start switching fruit for Snickers bars as your mid-morning snack, consider that the study was paid for by The Mars Corporation. Name ring a bell? How about The Mars

Candy Corporation? That's right, Mars, the makers of fine chocolate bars the world over, has funded this groundbreaking study on chocolate. How about "Payoff" for the name of their next candy bar?

THE BLAME GAME

There is a mindset that exists among people who battle lifelong weight problems which is very important to identify. It goes like this. Everything would be perfect in life if I just could lose the weight! My problem here is with the word "just." Being a thin person is a great way to get up in the morning, but it does not fix all of life's problems. I'll admit that my weight negatively affected my existence from childhood through my mid 30s, but like so many others, I pinned the answers to all of my money problems, relationship problems, career problems and family problems on my weight. I made the mistake of not trying to deal with or develop anything else in my life until I lost the weight. It's sort of like the struggling entertainer who puts off paying bills, doing taxes, making friends, getting married until he or she becomes a millionaire superstar. The entertainer, of course, never develops a quality life along the way and cannot obtain one by simply becoming a celebrity. Eventually, when they've achieved their lifelong goals and they take a good look around, they still feel empty about life. Hello, Betty Ford Center.

Overweight folks all too often do the same thing. They wait until they are thin to put together a quality life. I grew up thinking that suddenly when I lost the weight, all of my problems would magically go away. People would kiss my feet. The floodgates of opportunity would open and suddenly I'd be on easy street, be good at everything, and know everything about everything. Life would be pretty darned perfect.

I actually thought this way while growing up. Along the way, I noticed the same mindset in other people. Looking in the rearview mirror, I think it was a combination of thinking that the grass would always be greener if I was fit, and years of people telling me how much better life would be if I could just lose the weight. Imagine a youth filled with people taking you aside for one-on-one pep talks. Everyone you come into contact with—from mothers, fathers, sisters, brothers, grandparents, to teachers, friends, enemies, idols, girlfriends, doctors, acquaintances, household pets, strangers on the street, and even other heavy set people who actually thought they were thin—were all constantly telling you how much better you would feel and how much better your life would be if you could just get thin. *Get thin!* The desperation I placed upon those words became a true rallying cry.

I'll never get a chance to live my life over as the thin person I always wanted to be. I'm not even sure I'd want to if I could. The truth is, life is hard. It's a test. I don't need to be 165 pounds to ace it; I just need to be healthy enough to deal with its challenges. The Blame Game is a dangerous misconception. When I was 17 and 25 years old, I actually briefly achieved my goal weights. Blink and you missed it, but I actually *got thin.* It was anti-climatic, actually, because I'd set myself up for disappointment from the beginning. *Don't* let this happen to you.

Here's what I think you can count on if you are lucky enough to achieve your goal weight some day:

1. **You'll look more attractive and healthy.**

2. **You'll rid yourself of the weight discrimination and ridicule that infests our society.**

3. **You'll be able to think more clearly and be able to handle life's ups & downs easier.**

4. **You'll avoid the inevitable health problems that being overweight brings, such as heart attacks, strokes, type 2 diabetes, elevated blood pressure and sleep apnea.**

5. **You'll be more in control of your life.**

6. **You'll buy clothes off the rack.**

7. **You will not demolish lawn furniture like a crash-test dummy.**

8. **You will stop stressing out everyone who cares about you.**

9. **You will not avoid high school reunions.**

10. **You will live a better life, emotionally and physically.**

That's it. You'll still have bad days. You'll still need to learn. You'll still have to work through your other issues. People will still try to take advantage of you, and relationships will still require work. Money will still have to be earned. Also, on a personal note for you overweight guys out there, women will not kiss your feet when you've finally lost the weight. They will, however, stop blowing cigarette smoke in your face, and they may make eye contact and occasionally even give you their numbers. The truth is, if you are pinning your entire future on conquering food addiction, you are setting yourself up for a very big disappointment. A big fall. I've been there. I blamed all of my problems on my weight and when I eliminated the problem, my life was not exactly always wonderful, but it was a hell of a lot better. A major obstacle to finding happiness had been eliminated, but there was still a good deal of work to be done. It was simply a better "GO" point than where I was at before. A far better one. Don't set yourself up for disappointment. Know that you'll need to be physically and mentally healthy to deal with the things in life that will undoubtedly come at you. Get into the mindset of working on the other dreams you have for yourself. Improve all areas of your life while you are working on your health, because not everything depends on achieving the buff form you want. It's time to honestly evaluate your life. Which things in life are truly negatively affected by your weight, and which ones are not? My suggestion would be to start working on the things that aren't, because they'll still be there when you're healthy. As my brother Rich once so wisely put it, "The road to success is always under construction."

RELAPSE REDUX

Christmas, 2001. Harmon-Marino was producing events and holiday parties almost nightly. When there weren't company events, there were Christmas get-togethers with friends and family. At these functions there are endless buffets, some using an actual dream team of celebrity chefs like Todd English, Michael Schlow and Jasper White. Even though I tried staying on a healthy track, it was personally not a good time to be in the event business. By mid-December I was chasing down calzone with eggnog. It was in another free fall. *Lobster ravioli...hello. Pumpkin tortellini...are you kidding me? Mocha Marble Cheese Cake with white chocolate chips and strawberries...I'm about to lose control and I think I like it...*

This disease is incredible. I will always be amazed at how hard it is to stay on a healthy eating regimen, how quickly my bad habits come back, and how quickly I can fall back into "All" mode again. The old me is never far behind and the food is always so damn good. My mindset, at that time in 2001 (between appetizers of boneless honey BBQ chicken fingers and shrimp cocktails), I wished I could be an alcoholic. Let's face it, somehow today it's more respectable to be addicted to booze than burgers. Obviously, drug addicts and alcoholics have an awful disease too, but alas, they are not addicted to something you need to do three times every single day. On the other hand, as my comedian friend Tony V. once said, "I never threw a punch at my best friend over a blueberry pie."

The parties just kept coming, one more outrageous than the next. And there it was, the old me back just in time for the 2001 Christmas season. There was one major difference, however. I continued walking every day, knowing damn well that I won't be losing any weight. I seriously doubted that walking at this point would even help me keep from gaining weight, nor did I care. The new year was just around the corner and soon enough it would be time to begin eating healthy again. I had no desire to live the rest of my life an overweight, calzone-eating, eggnog-drinking putz. "There is more to life than food," I continued to tell myself. I don't know what ups and downs life has in store for me, but whatever they may be, I'm ready for them, good or bad, *if* I have my health.

◆   ◆   ◆

New Year's Eve. A time of reflection and renewal. No New Year's resolution is needed this year; I'm already fired up. I'm ready to get back on my weight loss routine when devastating news arrives. My brother's only child, my Godchild, Isabella Rose, suddenly died. Four-and-a-half years old and it's over. The family is numb. Inconsolable. Shocked. I rush to the side of my brother and his wife to try to help get them through the worst days of their lives. I've got to stay strong for everyone, to help lift the weight of that sadness. Still, the little angel is gone and it hurts. In between meetings with the priest, the funeral home and the cemetery, my eating goes from bad to worse. My brother's house is overdosed with lasagnas, cold cut platters, pies, donuts and chicken casseroles from well-meaning friends and family. I wish I could somehow funnel my pain into walks and healthy meals, but I can't. I feel awful. The pit in my stomach is the size of Ground Zero, and the devastated looks on everyone's faces only make me reach for yet another pastry.

Ahhh, pastry! For a split second it makes me feel better, and boy do I need my drug right now. It's three days until the funeral and every counter top and table is stacked with foil containers. I'm in a freefall. A typical day for me goes coffee, pastry, apple pie, some assorted nuts, salad, chicken Marsala, more apple pie (a la mode this time), tortellini in red sauce, Chinese food, tortellini in white sauce, antipasto (I'm pro-pasto myself) and Italian cold cut sandwiches. You get the picture. Post-traumatic Stretch Disorder is occurring and the daily overdose of food is only making me feel worse. I want my niece back. Her parents need their little girl back. No one should ever have to go through that type of pain. The kid crashed the planet when she arrived and everyone is wrecked by her unforeseen departure.

After the burial, I return home for the first time in a week, aware that I'm coming off of the worst month in my recovery so far. Somehow, somewhere, I've got to get off this funk train and back on my road to health. I'm desperate. I know I can undo everything I've accomplished in fairly short order if this downward spiral continues. Got to find some inspiration and get exercising again.

Sitting on the edge of my bed, I find myself staring at my departed niece's Christmas gift to me. She'd given me neck and ear warmers to wear on my walks. I had forgotten all about them in the devastation of the past week. I reached for them and headed for the lake. For the first time in two weeks, I was exercising again. My beautiful niece had inspired me to put an end to the self-destruction. A guy never could have asked for a better Godchild.

As I walked the lake that afternoon, a heavenly calm came over me. "I'm gonna be all right," I told myself. "I'm gonna be all right."

YOU'RE MY EVEREST

Some people are put on this planet to do great things: win the Olympics, write best sellers, make people laugh in movies, discover cures for terminal diseases, climb Mount Everest and inspire people to climb their own personal Everests. But how does someone accomplish great things when his obstacle in life is a giant mountain of buttery garlic mashed potatoes?

It's a tough world, folks. Even during the intense days of my recovery in 2001, detailed in the earlier chapters of this book, I was never able to fully stay on a healthy eating roll for more than five or six days. The weight came off slowly—painfully slowly. Sometimes it didn't come off at all. Now I was actually slipping the other way. 350 pounds was now pinching 360. What does one learn from this? That after 18 years of mental and financial torture, followed by two years of intense therapy with Ruth, while seeing a nutritionist like Melinda, walking almost daily and spending countless dollars to fix myself, I still could not gain control of my physical health. After everything I had been through, my life was still like a Ferrari with four flat tires. I was still just another overweight man in America and food addiction was no easier at 36 years of age than it was at 16, my friends.

In light of these feelings of hopelessness, my therapist Ruth and I got together for a spirited discussion in her office. These were never relationship-ending arguments, just spirited debates as to how to achieve the serenity and happiness that escaped me for what seemed like an eternity. At these debates, it always became apparent that I'd been connected to food since long before I could remember. My powerful, yet negative approach to food had created habits that were not easy to break. At therapy, Ruth explained to me that my connection to food went back to my early childhood, probably long before we were ripping up Mrs. Harrigan's lawn playing football. My love for food developed at a very young age and only became more intense as my childhood progressed into adulthood. The Feedback Cycle (the continual pleasure a young child derives from food) began. Then she dropped a bombshell on me. Ruth revealed to me that in all her years as a therapist who specializes in weight issues, she never knew anyone who has beaten this illness for any sustained amount of time. Never, in over twenty years of practicing, had she personally seen anyone beat this disease, with the exception of those who have undergone radical stomach bypass surgery or made it through the intensity of Overeaters Anonymous. Stop the presses! The harshness of her revelation came crashing down on me like a ton of bacon. Beating this disease was going to be an odds-defying and daunting task. I'd already ruled out both the surgery and OA unless the day came when I couldn't get out of bed. That's the solemn promise I'd made to myself. Now, as I sat there in therapy land with Ruth, it began to dawn on me that I'd only scraped the surface of this problem. Everything I'd done up to then was simply preparation and education for a ground war, an offensive which would demand a massive effort if I was going to achieve victory. Ruth was not trying to discourage me in any way. She was simply leveling with me about the task I was attempting and how difficult it actually was.

Sitting in her office, I was actually in awe of what had just been realized. At this point Ruth was still talking to me and I was not even listening anymore. I barely heard a word of what she was saying to me. And in my mind's eye, at that very moment I was standing at the foot of a massive mountain, which was my disease.

I do not know why this disease was thrust upon me, but it's my life's challenge to defeat it. I have only just begun to fight, and I swear as I sit here today, I will be victorious. I do not care how long it takes. And I'm staring up intensely at you, my old nemesis. Coming at you with guns blazing. It may take a lifetime, but I'm going to conquer you. YOU'RE MY EVEREST.

INTENSITY vs MAKESENSITY

Getting back into the groove has always been a problem for me. I think it is for most people who struggle with their weight. It's the Monday Morning Dieter Syndrome. It's cutting off the feedback cycle. Breaking up with a girlfriend whom you love, but who you know will ruin you. By the time I had dropped 60 pounds or so in the winter of 2002, I'd realized that my approach to getting back to losing weight and exercising had always been too jarring and too intense—a jolt to the mind and body which left me essentially detoxing and feeling denied.

Every Sunday night I'd stuff the rest of the lasagna down at 10:00 p.m. so I could hit the fresh yogurt and strawberries by 8:00 a.m. Monday. Cold turkey. Sometimes the intensity of jumping back into a healthy lifestyle can trip you up. It's a delicate process, learning to love and then to miss that light, healthy feeling. It starts by slowly introducing good foods and punctual eating times back into your day. After three or four days, when you're feeling good again, you're ready to reintroduce exercise back into your life. Maybe not six or seven days a week, but two or three at first. The eye of the tiger, or what's today referred to as "the zone," is one and a half to two weeks away. Grab it when you can and hold on for dear life. These are the times when you can make some real headway. Realizing just how precious these spurts of healthy eating and exercising are is invaluable to your success. Now fit individuals may exercise and eat properly every day and not have to think much about it. Then again, those same people could probably never imagine looking at a Chinese food combo platter and saying "You're my Everest" either. They are just two different existences. Unfortunately, we need a little more of what they've got, which is balance, discipline and self-control.

In an effort to try to achieve a little of that balance, discipline and self-control, I introduced a new trick to my growing arsenal of healthy tools. Anyone I'd ever met in my life who beat this disease had always described the process as learning to play the piano or riding a bike. I guess this new routine fell into that category. Each week, beginning on Sunday or Monday, I looked at my calendar for the week ahead and take note of what was on my work and social schedules. I identified "Impeccable Days," which were days when I had nothing but work on my calendar, and "Maintenance Days," which were days when I was meeting a client for lunch or dinner or producing an event at work involving a Jurassic-Park-sized buffet. I considered "Impeccable Days" as days of opportunity; a productive time period to be seized for weight loss purposes. In my mind, there was no reason whatsoever to falter on those days. Walking and eating a low-calorie, low-carb regimen was gospel, so the only thing stopping me on these days was me. I, at this point in my life, was strong enough to battle my inner demons.

Frankly, I'd had enough of my inner voice giving in every time I smelled Chinese food outside of my car window. I knew that whenever I was in that moment, arguing with myself about whether I should or shouldn't, the person who wanted a happy, healthy lifestyle, would win. Impeccable days were also days when the selfish person (the one who needs to be in all of us to put ourselves first) would come out. No one was going to convince me to break my healthy routine on these days.

Maintenance Days, on the other hand, were treat days, times when I knew I wouldn't be losing weight. But there was absolutely no reason to gain weight, thereby reversing all of the work I'd done, for some cheap love from a fast food place. That approach made no sense to me anymore. If I had a Maintenance Day scheduled, it was usually because I was going to a great restaurant or working in what Ruth called a "perverse situation," such as a resort with outrageous food. I enjoyed the food, but I would just not go off on it. No denial, but no free-for-all either. I knew the next day I would not have lost weight, but I also realized that I had maintained my previous weight loss and still enjoyed the lure of delicious food. I was in control. There was also a major change in these situations. The All-or-Nothing Syndrome was no longer around. I'd retired that addictive behavior for the betterment of my existence.

The hopeless food addict I once was would look at a Maintenance Day—let's say a dinner with a friend in Boston's North End (our version of Little Italy)—as an All Day. The addict mindset would be *Screw it all. I'm not going to lose weight anyway after a 5-course meal and lots of wine, so why not enjoy a great breakfast and try that new lunch place as well? Get it all in today, you're in a free-for-all!*

The new me had a much more sensible approach. For example, I would take it easy during the day. Breakfast and lunch resembled my Impeccable Day regimen. I knew I'd enjoy that evening's food and wine a hell of a lot more if I wasn't bloated and stuffed upon my arrival, and I'd probably be a lot better company if I weren't pumping gas into a gas tank that was already full. With my old all-or-nothing approach, I gained weight the next day. Three overdone meals and no exercise equals weight gain, essentially undoing the precious work that had already been done. With my new approach (Maintenance Days), I'd have an impeccable weight loss day and then be able to slip some of my old friends in the back door—old friends like steak fries, garlic-mashed potatoes, Chinese food, ribs, ribs, ribs, etc. Before I could feel badly about indulging my old demons, I'd be back to walking 6 miles again. Instead of falling back into my comfortably numb ways, I'd already be back achieving true happiness, feeling good about my body.

R.I.P. All or Nothing

1976-2001.

The Art Of
THE SALAD BAR

Recovering from a lifetime of food addiction is never a quick and easy process. It takes time to recondition your thinking and to educate yourself about nutrition. It also means you have to learn to take a second look at situations that seemed healthy only yesterday. One example is the good old-fashioned Salad Bar. Just when you think you're being good, you may have gone over to the dark side without even realizing it.

It all starts innocently enough. You enter a restaurant and follow the hostess to your seat, with every intention of being good. On the way to your table you pass a long and colorful salad bar. "I think I'll eat healthy today," you tell yourself. "Besides, I'll spend less money." When the waitress approaches you a minute later with menus and specials, you cut her off in mid-sentence and proudly declare, "I'll just do the Salad Bar." Your dinner guests are impressed with your new healthy attitude, and decide to be supportive and join you, even though you know that if you had their bodies, you'd be ordering the "All the beef ribs you can eat" special.

You approach the salad buffet and grab a plate, immediately noticing how fresh, crisp and piled high everything is. Just eyeing that baby makes you feel good about yourself, doesn't it? You begin laying down a nice bed of salad greens as your foundation, maybe some Iceberg here, a little Romaine there. You then add eight or ten fresh cherry tomatoes, perhaps even popping one in your mouth like a piece of candy. Sweet. A little further up you add some cucumber wedges, red onion slices and cuts of yellow pepper. Nice. The weight-loss gods are smiling down on you at this point. Then something catches your eye that sends things in the wrong direction. *Are those green olives?* You've heard they weren't the best for you, something about the fat content. You decide a few green olives can't take down an entire salad, so you scoop half a dozen or so of those babies onto your plate, and then go back for a second scoop to round it out to a dozen. As you're about to move on, you notice that next to the green olives is a mountain of black ones. You've got to have variety, right? So you add a dozen of those as well. Shredded cheddar cheeses are next up, and you decide that if you're going to have that many olives, a little cheddar won't hurt either. The bacon bits are located next to the cheddar, and you put just half a scoop on your salad, knowing you have to police yourself at some point. Chunks of Swiss cheese are neatly sliced into cubes just a little further down and you decide that since you're not being a total purist with your salad, a few of those won't hurt either. Next, a bin of hard-boiled eggs comes into view, and you tell yourself that there is still enough room on the sides of the plate to fit four or five. Besides, did you even eat breakfast today?

At this point you've crossed over to the dark side. The weight of the plate begins to become a problem, but that doesn't stop you from adding a scoop of tuna salad, a scoop of macaroni salad and maybe a scoop of potato salad. You pass on the scoop of egg salad because you are still trying to be good. Besides, you've already hit your egg quota with the hard-boiled variety. The crouton station is next. Although you've decided to knock off unnecessary breads, you know you've already crossed the line of being healthy somewhere back around the bacon bits. As you add the crunchy croutons to the heap, you notice that they are falling off the top of your plate with nothing to stick to. You'll need some good thick dressing to hold those babies up there, so you head over to the assorted salad dressings. There are enough croutons on the plate to give you a yeast infection, but all you care about is keeping them affixed to your salad. You know the vinaigrette dressing won't hold the croutons in place, as its consistency isn't quite thick enough. The low-calorie Italian doesn't appeal to you at this point, after all this stopped being about health ten minutes ago. The French dressing might hold croutons, but wait. Is that Blue Cheese? That'll do the trick. You grab the ladle and scoop it on. One scoop for the croutons. Once they're firmly secured, another scoop for the top layers of your giant salad, If we can even call it that now. Just in case the lower sections (the iceberg and romaine layers) are still dry, you throw a third scoop on, hoping it will eventually find it's way down. As you reach the end of the buffet, you notice your cohorts adding spaghetti and clam chowder to their plates, but there's no real estate left on yours this trip. With cherry tomatoes rolling off, you head to the cash register, where a cashier struggles to lift the produce Everest onto the scale.

"14 dollars and 33 cents," she declares without making eye contact. So much for cheap. So much for health. If her scale could measure calories, you'd land somewhere around the 3,000 range.

Sound familiar? If not, try this one on for size. You're at a yogurt shop. You eyeball the flavors warily, because you want to keep it healthy. You ask the clerk for a sample of the fat-free Dutch Apple yogurt. It's good, but you're not sold on it. "How many calories in the Peach?" you ask, requesting another sample. As you try it, you notice that the Dutch Apple is still on your taste buds, so you try another just to get the flavor. No go. "Is the White Chocolate sugar free?" you inquire.

"Yes, sir," says the Doogie Howser-looking kid behind the counter.

"Okay, give me a large fat-free, sugar-free White Chocolate with crushed Oreo cookies and chunks of Snickers bars on top."

Ah, America, the land of opportunity and calories! If you're struggling with your weight, you may want to avoid perverse situations. These include salad buffets, breakfast buffets, Chinese food buffets, the "Super" buffet, the Old Country buffet, the Jimmy Buffett buffet, and the Eat-Till-You-Implode Buffet. They are all wonderful and we are lucky to live in a country where food is so readily available, but if food is your drug, sheer abundance can become the enemy. Comedian Robin Williams once described cocaine as "God's way of telling you you're making too much money." In my opinion, buffets are God's way of telling folks they've got way too much time on their hands. Do we really need five types of potatoes prepared five different ways? Now I can't even begin to say "hello" to a buffet until I've filled three or four plates, but here is a way to handle a buffet if you must put yourself in the same room with one. In Melinda's opinion, salad bars can be your best friend or your worst enemy. Here are her suggestions on keeping the nutrition count high and the calorie count low.

MELINDA'S GUIDE TO HEALTHY EATING AT SALAD BARS

If you are trying to eat a salad as a meal, the goal is quite different than having one as a side.

For a meal, you want to make that salad as "balanced" as possible. In other words, you should identify a carbohydrate source, a fat source and a protein source. Next, you want those sources to be as healthy as possible, given what your choices are. Here are some examples:

Healthy carbohydrate sources

Vegetables. All vegetables are carbs, but you can be fooled if they are swimming in lots of fat, like dressings or marinades, so try to stick with the plain veggies and dress them yourself with the available dressings. Vegetables that have deep colors like green, red, orange, yellow, or blue/purple tend to give you more nutrients than white veggies. Choose more colors for nutrition and avoid "fillers" like iceburg lettuce and skinless cucumbers (unless you want the filler to help you get full). By the way, it is ok to choose some "starchy" veggies like corn and peas, as these contribute good nutrients to a meal plan, just watch the portion.

Potatoes are ok unless they are slathered in mayo, oils, etc. In that case, you are getting a whole lot more than you bargained for.

Legumes. Yes, beans are a "good" carb source, and guess what? They also make a decent protein source as well, and one that is chock full of fiber to boot.

Nuts and Seeds. These not only make a good carb choice, but also contribute a very healthy fat source as well.

Cheese. Believe it or not, cheese—including cottage cheese, mozzarella, and feta cheeses—are a better source of carbs than they are protein. But remember to use these in moderation, as most cheeses on the salad bar contain a sizeable amount of fat and so carry a lot of weight, so to speak.

The carbohydrates that you should be careful with are the rice, pasta, and other grain salads. Often, they are floating in oily dressings or mayonnaise and contribute a large amount of carbohydrates, compared to a relatively small amount in the above choices.

Healthy Protein Choices

Of course the obvious choices are turkey breast meat, chicken breast and tuna (preferably not in mayo, but plain). Other fair choices can be ham, or small amounts of cheese like mozzarella or feta. Unfortunately, cheese is a much better source of unhealthy fat (saturated fat) than it is protein, so use it sparingly. Cottage cheese is a wonderful source of protein with less fat content than most cheeses.

My favorite, of course, are legumes. Legumes, in my opinion, are one of the most perfect foods, and they lend texture and flavor to any dish. Beans, such as kidney beans, chickpeas, red beans, black beans, black-eyed peas, etc., are great sources of fiber and a fair source of protein (not to mention carbs). Legumes are an almost perfectly-balanced food.

Healthy Fat Sources

The fats to include, in moderation, are the vegetable oils. Some of the favorites, especially in adding flavor, are olive oil, nut oils, and seed oils. Just remember that every tablespoon of oil is adding an extra 100 calories to your salad! So pour carefully, and drain veggies that come dressed. Nuts and seeds, as mentioned above, contribute a little of everything, but especially a lot of heart-healthy fat. Olives, green or black, in very small quantities contribute very healthy fat and add good flavor to salads.

Avoid, if possible, cream-based dressings, foods that come in mayonnaise-based dressings, bacon bits, lots of cheeses, etc. Vinegar is fine to use, and virtually calorie free.

To sum up:

Choose lots of plain vegetables that have good, deep, rich color. Choose moderate amounts of lean protein choices. Choose very small amounts of fat choices.

MY BODY THE TEMPLE:
Feeling the low-carb love

March 2002. What a time to be alive! New England was experiencing its warmest winter in 135 years. The New England Patriots were Super Bowl Champions. I was back walking four to six miles per day and feeling really good again. Ah, that light feeling those fit and trim folks seemed to live for. I was slowly beginning to understand. As a matter of fact, I was as addicted to feeling light on my feet as I ever was to feeling a cheeseburger in my hands. If this was how 39% of the country lived, I liked their style. After flunking a pop quiz in a men's health magazine, I decided it might be time to up the ante a bit. The test asked the following question:

Which of these activities burns the most calories?

(A) Walking (B) Swimming (C) Weight Training

Naturally, I wanted the answer to be my exercise of choice, which was walking. But based on the sticky numbers on the scale each week, I circled swimming, figuring it used the entire body and would maximize calorie burning. To my surprise, the answer was weight training, and it instantly got my attention. Early in my recovery I ruled out lifting weights, based on every doctor I'd ever known telling me I'd only be building fat. "Get the weight off first, then build your body into muscle," they said, but like everything else in the health business, that advice went the way of the dieting concept. Thanks to the Bulldog back in the 1970s, I didn't need much convincing to stay away from anything painful, such as lifting weights. It had been 22 years since I'd joined a gym as a serious member. Jimmy Carter was President. Richard Simmons barely even had a career going. Nevertheless, the new theory among professionals was that it was the way to go, no matter how much you weighed.

Intrigued, I decided to add a new member to the dream team. This time it was a fitness trainer named Vincent Zarella. My friend and mortgage broker Bob Devasto recommended him to me over lunch one day. Within 48 hours, Vincent was standing in my office. He was young, smart and a real character. The kid's body was a rock and we instantly hit it off. We commenced working out together in the spring at RMA Fitness in Wilmington. It wasn't all that convenient for me in terms of location, but it was clearly time to kick my physical game into high gear, so on Tuesdays and Thursdays I headed up to the RMA to take the physical part of my recovery from decaf to speedball.

Both Dr. Zarins and Melinda suspected that my daily five and six mile walks were not having as much impact on my weight loss situation as they had a year and a half earlier. It was hard to believe, but aside from burning calories, which was always good, my body had become conditioned to the walks. My heart rate wasn't getting high enough, the process of burning fat was not happening, and therefore it was time to begin intensifying my workouts. That's where Vincent came in.

The first day was simply classic. There Vincent and I were, in a worn down section of the gym, doing stretches and getting to know each other. "You can call me the Vin Man if you like," he said. Now that alone would have sent the old me running for the door.

"First we'll work on your glutes," the Vin Man said.

"Glutes? Where's that?" I asked. Vincent pointed to my lower butt cheeks. "You mean, like, my assticular muscles?" I joked.

"We should do some exercises for your obliques, too," he suggested. Now I had absolutely no idea where the obliques were, but I suspected mine were pretty, well, bleak. "That sounds good," I responded enthusiastically.

As was my signature trademark, I was serving up the self-deprecating humor large, but Vincent just smirked and kept it all business. I explained to him that this was the first gym I'd worked out in since 1980. Maybe that's when he knew what he was up against. Our typical workout in those days involved a 15-minute warm-up on the treadmill, followed by 10 minutes of intense stretching exercises. How intense? Well, when you get winded from stretching, you know it's intense. Following that, Vincent ran me through every routine from free weights to Cybex machines to step aerobics. We did three sets each of leg press, bench press, seated rows, and bicep curls. Between routines, while Vincent put the appropriate weights on and adjusted the machines, he had me doing step-ups or other routines designed to keep my heart rate high during the workouts. Twenty-two years later, I was still not a fan of self-induced pain, but in time, I began to adjust and learn to look forward to "the burn," as my brothers out on the mats say.

And that wasn't the only adjusting going on. Melinda and I continued to tweak and adjust my way-of-life eating plan, and it began to look like the perfect marriage of a good old-fashioned low-calorie regimen combined with an "Atkins Lite" type program. I wasn't going overboard on the protein and meats, but I was definitely backing off big time on the breads and whites. By that time the Atkins diet was the rage in America, but Melinda was shrewd enough to know it wasn't for me. First, because it simply wasn't meant for someone with 200 pounds to lose. Second, why force the possibility of high cholesterol or high blood pressure on a body that didn't have those problems?

On the positive side, it was amazing how good I felt once I'd eliminated such carbohydrate overdoses as garlic mashed potatoes, Portuguese sweet rolls, pasta, and of course my old personal favorite, Killer Bread. I'd learned how to make Killer Bread during my days as a cook in Marco Island, and it became my version of cocaine. To make it, you basically took a large slice of Italian bread grilled in garlic butter and spread it with a deadly combination of Parmesan cheese and mayonnaise.

Is your mouth watering yet? Don't get all hot and bothered. It's hardly worth the deadly assault on your heart. And on a personal note, for me nothing was worth what I went through. For me, Killer bread equaled a Killer weight problem, one that I was finally beginning to take control of, perhaps for the first time in my life.

By the time I'd hit 335 pounds in April of 2002, something strange had begun happening. Convinced that I was on my way to being healthy again (for the first time in over a decade), I was becoming very protective of which foods I put in my body. Fast foods and desserts like cheesecake were beginning to look like the devil. When someone offered me anything even remotely like that, I'd stare at it repulsively, like an old enemy whose game I was hip to. I resented what foods like that had done to my life and what little benefit my body could reap from their contents. I'd become pretty darned protective of what exactly I would put in my body, which was a far cry from the kamikaze eater I'd been through my teens, 20s and the first half of my 30s. At steak restaurants, where the cooks were known to put ladles of butter directly on the meat or grilled vegetables, I ordered my meal with "absolutely no butter." My stern attitude always prompted the waitress to ask, "Do you have some sort of reaction to butter, sir?"

"Yes, it makes me fat," I answered with a smile.

I'd been reading and studying about nutrition every day by this point, and was slowly beginning to understand exactly how and why the American diet had gone wrong, and how it had resulted in the country now being a staggering 61% overweight.

Sugars. Complex carbohydrates. Fat grams. Saturated fats. Up until now I had only been aware of calories per serving. The more I read, the more I began seeing myself as a grown up statistic. Slowly I was becoming that anal retentive big guy you occasionally see in the supermarket, holding up traffic in the cereal isle so he can compare a box of Cheerios to a box of Wheaties on calories and sugars. *Don't rush me folks, my body is a temple.*

Besides reading every box for nutrition facts, I began to frequent restaurants dedicated to the art of serving what a healthy human body needed. Eateries who listed the calories and carbs right on their menus. Places where a guy struggling to regain control of his health could find a great meal without the guilt. On any given weekday you'd find me at Lo Fat Know Fat High Protein Low Carb Grille & Café in Watertown, Mass. They served tasty sandwiches such as chicken meatball, veggie burritos, and Bison Burger Wraps. The concept, founded by Tim Kurtz and Chris Pappas, was the first of its kind in the area. It was very liberating to eat at Lo Fat Know Fat with clients or friends and not have to worry about walking into a perverse atmosphere. Walk in healthy, walk out healthy. What a concept! The folks at Lo Fat Know Fat had another novel concept going which excited me: air fries. As in french fries, prepared in a hot air oven versus a traditional deep fry-o-later. By 2002, french fries were the number one vegetable consumed in the United States, but to most folks—myself included—potatoes ceased to be vegetables after they took a swan dive into a pool of deep frying oil set at 360 degrees. In addition to air fries, Lo Fat Know Fat stocked a massive variety of healthy desserts, protein bars, meal replacement products and fitness magazines.

I was also, at this time, opening up to the concept of raw and organic foods, and my brother Rich, 39 years old and now firmly entrenched in his own weight problem, was convinced that raw foods were the answer to true and lasting health. But could uncooked foods ever actually be delicious? Would the masses open up to eating anything that wasn't cooked in a fryolator? Rich was a man on a mission to find out, and who better than a guy who owned and operated a successful gourmet Italian restaurant? Chianti Tuscan Grill had been open since 1992 in Beverly, MA, and it's loyal following made it one of the North Shore's premiere restaurants.

Perhaps spurred on by his need of an outlet after his daughter's recent death, or by my lifelong battle with weight (and now perhaps even his own), Rich began experimenting with the concept of gourmet Italian food dishes that were low calorie, low carbohydrate and very low in fat. Revolutionary! Pasta dishes without the pasta. Cream sauces without the cream. His ideas were so brilliant and well-intentioned that I quickly began incorporating them into my daily regimen. Guess what? I continued losing three to six pounds per month. Move over, Subway Sandwiches! A couple of overweight Italian boys from Boston may have just stumbled onto something here. Something real.

I've Relapsed Again...And I Can't Get Up!

"Humble pie is extremely low in calories"

—Author Unknown

Just when you thought we'd gotten to the part of the book where the subject fixes his problem and forges on to victory in a "Rocky III" type ending, guess what? This book is all about reality, folks. I may run out of chapter names using the word relapse, but I'll always seize the opportunity to prove that there is simply no easy way to fix a lifelong weight problem. It's the hardest thing to do in the world.

Late May, 2002. I'm not sure exactly what caused it this time. Maybe it was my discouragement at losing only three pounds for the entire month of April, which had been one of the best months I'd ever had in terms of exercising and eating healthy. Perhaps it was emotional derailment. My niece was gone and her parents needed us to help them get through the depressing days. My business was a disorganized mess. A runaway train, which was stressing me out beyond belief. My marriage to Julie was beginning to feel the ill effects of everything, which only added to my emotional distress. Another possible scenario for the relapse that made sense was the fact that I was attempting to lose weight without the help of drugs like Meridia and Xenical, or surgeries such as Gastric Bypass and Gastric Band Implantation. It was all becoming too much. I was at war with myself and it was getting to me. The Ben & Jerry's Chunky Monkey was on my back once again (I'm polishing off a pint as I write this. No joke).

One night in early June, Julie and I took my niece Mackenzie to the Rainforest Cafe in Burlington. I, of course, was back in "All" mode again. Due to my excessive work schedule, I hadn't walked in two weeks. Mackenzie ordered pasta with red sauce, while I ordered the Ribs, Chimi Changas and Coconut Chicken—you know, in case the kid wanted a little extra something to snack on. You can never be too sure in these troubled times, can you? That bloated, sedated feeling had returned and I was feeling ugly. That aura of burning rubber was back again, which only made me want to eat more. "Sometimes I swear the only difference between me and the crack addict over there in the alley is that my needle says "Ben & Jerry's," I half-heartedly joked with my wife.

As I fell back into my "All or Nothing" food funk, my priorities, as they had my whole life, became twisted. In early June my photographer friend Leo Gozbekian asked if I wanted to do a meet-and-greet with the singer Alanis Morrisette backstage at a show in Mansfield MA. Her album, *Jagged Little Pill*, was one of the 90s best sellers and today it's still a classic. Matty Blake, one of my comedian clients, and I arrived at the backstage area about five minutes before show time. It was 8:20 p.m. and I hadn't eaten yet. There was only enough time to get a bite to eat or to meet Alanis. Meet the superstar or eat? Eat or meet the superstar? If I hadn't been relapsing at this point, I'd have loved to meet this Jagged Little Pill. But naturally, the Jagged Little Sausage Stand won out and got the best of me. *Maybe I'll say hello after the concert*, I quickly reasoned with myself. Relapsing is pathetic. But you know what? It's okay. Relapsing is a reality for the rest of your life if you're trying to lose weight and keep it off. Don't beat yourself up and throw in the towel. That's what I told myself, anyway.

So, after a year and a half, several thousand dollars and countless hours of effort, it was time to get serious. The United States was on a heightened state of alert from terrorists, and I was on a heightened state of alert from Tiramisu. I would not spend another minute relapsing in some Chimi Changa coma. My life was passing me by and I was still eating and wanting to gorge myself, and in turn it was eating away at me. So what do you do when you've given it an honest effort, recruited the best minds in the business and still failed to achieve true health? Roll the dice, go for broke and pull out all of the stops, right?

In June of 2002 I closed my office in Burlington, MA, let go of my office help and reduced Harmon-Marino Entertainment to a virtual business being run via cell phone and laptop computer. As I've said, the company hadn't grown the way I'd hoped it would. Physically, mentally and spiritually I was ripping down the shack at the bottom of the hill so I could build the mansion on top of the hill. Why rip down what I had worked so hard to build? Because work was stressing me out, which only made me want to eat. The overhead of a 1,000-square-foot office, couriers, computers, cameramen, the administrative assistant, the accountant, the lawyer, utilities, dumpster fees, etc. was stressing me out, which only made me want to eat. And finally, a work schedule of 60-plus hours per week, multiple projects and shows all with their own set of details and all at various stages of completion was keeping me from exercising. That in turn only made me want to eat. It's a two-part process—exercising and eating—right? It's 50/50. You can't truly do one without the other, so I decided that after 10 years of trying to build a successful business I'd concentrate on building a successful human first. Physical health, followed by mental health. A complete re-inventing of myself while in my middle to late thirties. In addition, I also jettisoned some longtime personal and business friendships. As hard as it was, it was the right move to make. Drastic times call for drastic measures. People who drain your batteries, even if they are good people, can stress you out and sabotage your health. Surround yourself with too many of these types of people and you can lose yourself. For the first time in my life, I was putting myself first. My mom had always talked about putting myself first. In order to do that I had to lighten my workload, lower my overhead, and make myself socially scarce. Her death convinced me to shift priorities in a way I never thought I would have to. As a result, my career was about to take a serious back seat. And if Harmon-Marino didn't survive? Then so be it. As long as I had my health, I was convinced that I could build a new life and maybe even a better career. I decided I'd embargo all of my free time detoxing myself with a stricter food regimen (compliments of Melinda), and sandwiching my days between swimming laps in the pool every morning and walking five to six miles every afternoon. I rolled with my faith in God, the future, and myself and stepped up to the highway to health, which by this time I had nicknamed "The Million Calorie March."

◆　　◆　　◆

It wasn't easy, but by late July I was back on my game in terms of health. Working out with my trainer, Vincent, I was beginning to understand the meaning of the saying "hurts so good." Up until now, I'd only equated working out with the word "hurt." Now *hurts so good* meant more to me than a John Mellencamp tune from the 80s. The scale was now reading 324 pounds. *Crack 300,* I thought, *and it's a whole new game.*

By late summer I had become another person and people were beginning to notice. My days were dedicated to exercise. I'd wake up around 7:00 a.m., walk into my new home office, check e-mails and voice mails, and then head for the gym or the lake. Vincent was working me incredibly hard and was excited about my progress. After a ten-minute workout on the treadmill, followed by 25 minutes on the cross-trainer, and then ten more minutes of stretches, he'd have me in the zone. During the intense workouts I'd get very serious and intense myself. "Do you feel okay?" the Vin Man would ask.

"Don't let the palpable tension fool you, my friend," I'd respond. "I am loving this pain."

In between some intense weight-lifting, Vincent had me doing pushups, sit-ups, step-ups and medicine ball tosses, right there in the middle of the gym for everyone to see. I was on a mission indeed. After the gym workouts I upped the ante with marathon walks. A heat wave of 90 degree weather, including downright unhealthy humidity, had gripped Massachusetts. However, I was undaunted. One day, with my cousin Michele—by now a weight loss soul mate—I walked the Charles River in Boston for a solid two and a half hours. Two days later, while in Cape Cod on business, I walked a bike path from Falmouth to Woods Hole. From there I walked several neighborhoods and private beaches before heading back down the bike path towards Falmouth: a total walking time of three hours. The following Monday I dropped my car off at a dealership in my hometown of Medford, handed my keys to the service girl and said, "Call me at home when it's done." Slightly confused, she asked me how I was getting home. "Walking," I responded.

"South Medford to Woburn? You're crazy!" Maybe I was, but I didn't care at that point. "I need it," I said as I jammed out the door. A total walking time of two hours and fifteen minutes. When I walked through the door that afternoon, the phone was ringing. "Mr. Marino, your car is all set to be picked up," said the voice on the other end of the line.

"Great," I said as I packed a towel and headed to the pool for some laps. There would, of course, be a price to pay for all of this exercise. I'd be in my little home office most nights paying for the downtime. In the gym the next day I was excited to jump on the scale, a ritual I usually reserved for Melinda; but Vincent was telling me all morning how well I was doing and how much my physical appearance had changed in the last three weeks. I was focused intensely on breaking 300, and figured that after the phenomenal week of exercise and eating right, I'd be somewhere in the 318 to 319 range. In the men's locker room I jumped on a digital scale. "335" said Vincent. I looked down in shock.

"No way! This thing is wrong!" I exploded.

Vincent, putting up no argument, calmly said, "Maybe it is; let's get you on the weight scale over here." 335 again. I started to flip out and Vincent put an immediate stop to it. "Let me jump on, let's see if my weight is correct." It was. I was horrified. I threw a tantrum in the gym that took Vincent several minutes to calm. I reserved judgment on the scale numbers until I saw Melinda two days later. As the numbers reached a mind-numbing 335 again on her scale, a fury began to rise deep within me. What had happened? What was I doing? Why was I walking miles outside of town everyday? Why was I spending money on trainers and nutritionists and therapists? All of this, and I had *gained* weight! I was disgusted. Melinda immediately went into "don't get discouraged" mode, but I was aghast by the possibility that I'd somehow gained 11 pounds during one of the most intense stretches of healthy eating and exercise in my entire life.

"What happened?" I asked Melinda desperately.

"I'm not sure exactly," she replied. "It could be a shift in body weight or the fat turning to muscle, but whatever you do, don't get discouraged." Discouraged? I was appalled! Why was I denying myself every day? To *gain* weight? Something was wrong when a 330-pound guy radically changed his food intake, as well as exercise, and gained weight. Once again, Melinda noted for me that most folks had lost and gained their weight back in the time it took me to lose 65 pounds. She reminded me that my resolve was still there throughout. Nevertheless, I left Melinda's office feeling extremely defeated and ready to settle the score. I'd been robbed of substantial weight loss and it became apparent that the weight loss gods were not shining on me. *Welcome to the real world, Son; you're on your own.*

JURASSIC PASTA:
When Bloated Things Happen To Good People

In late summer of 2002 I had an epiphany. Now to most health nuts and nutritionists it might not have seemed like much of a startling revelation, but to this lifelong food addict it was an epiphany of monumental proportions. It not only helped me to understand why I'd been struggling with a weight problem for an eternity, but it also helped me get one step closer to understanding why the weight wasn't coming off, even with the huge turn around I'd made in my mid-30s. I'd spent lots of time at libraries, bookstores and on the Internet, reading as much as I could about nutrition and weight loss. Yes, indeed, you could find me in the self-help section of fine bookstores all across New England.

I slowly began to realize what the human body needed: healthy eating vs. what entire generations had grown up to believing was normal eating; eating for what your body needed vs. your taste buds. I began to understand why everybody around me seemed to be struggling with their weight. Abundance had strangely become the enemy. People were overdosing on carbs, fats and calories and thinking it was normal eating because they'd been conditioned to believe so. It certainly made sense in my case. If you've been reading this, you all know by now where I've been. As I studied nutrition and what the body truly needed for fuel, I began to realize just how off course we were in America in 2002.

Movie theaters were selling jacuzzi-sized soft drinks. Gas stations had morphed into supermarkets selling tons of junk foods. *Fill 'er up and get me a cheese steak pocket.* Pizza makers were now blowing cheese into the pizza crust with some sort of semi-automatic cheese gun. As if pizza wasn't unhealthy enough, we now had to jam cheese into the crust? Stuffed quahogs were being made with chunks of linguica mixed in with the bread crumbs and butter. As a result, the texture was so thick it could be used for home improvement projects ranging from spackling walls to filling gaps in concrete.

Snack food vending machines, often located in schools, hospitals, and office complexes, offered anything but healthy products. Fifty to sixty food choices were available, yet the only items to pick from were M&Ms, Raisinets, Doritos, potato chips and the like. Not that we needed fresh pineapple chunks or soy nuts in there, but couldn't something healthy be offered? Where were items such as nuts, healthy meal-replacement bars, yogurt bars, or drinks without corn syrup?

In the dairy sections of supermarkets, "healthy yogurts" were sold with chocolate chips, chocolate-covered granola or sugary crunchies in plastic containers attached to the lids, which essentially cancelled out the healthy part. There's an answer to our country's *rampant thinness epidemic*, right? A healthy product packaged with an unhealthy companion. A right and a wrong in the same product does not make a right, but your average consumer with a few pounds to lose was throwing it on the conveyer belt to be "good." Food was all around people at any given time and everywhere they looked. "The land of plenty" had taken on a new and ominous meaning.

In fine Italian restaurants everywhere, folks were being served Jurassic portions of pasta as main courses, with cream sauces or red sauces, packed with more meat and spices than my Grandma LaCamera ever dreamed of. Americans were lapping it up. Call me crazy, but even the Statue Of Liberty was beginning to look a little bloated. The carbohydrate overdose was leaving people lethargic and inactive. I began noticing in restaurants just how sedated people were by food, sitting around in their food funks, looking as if someone had sucked the life out of them. I knew all too well how they felt. People dilated by food. Bloated into oblivion.

I began joking with friends and family about a future time when products listed Bloat Factors on their labels, much like sun block companies listed Sun Protection factors. *Does anyone want some Pecan Pie? Well, let's take a look. What's the Bloat Factor? 87 BF? I'd better back off. Say, what's the Bloat Factor on that 7 layer Mexican dip? 84? That's not bad.*

Of course, it wasn't just the types of food that put people in comas, it was the amounts they were consuming. Nowhere had it ever been said that eating large portions of those types of foods was what the human body needed, yet everywhere you looked, people were overdosing their bodies because they'd come to believe it was normal.

Donut shops were serving everything from giant scones to coconut custard and spiced apple-filled donuts. The sizes were twice the normal amount and twice the calories and sugars. *I'll have half a dozen Vanilla Crème donuts and a cholesterol test to go, please.*

Calzone places were going up everywhere with every type of filling imaginable: cold cut, spinach and cheese, chicken parmesan, and three cheese. *Could you please get on the other side of this steak and cheese calzone and help me carry it to my trunk?*

Breakfast places were serving eggs along with bacon, sausages, pancakes, corn beef hash and bagels in entrees with names such as "The Plantation" or "The Farmer's Breakfast." Now that may have been fine for the American farmer who plowed fields for ten hours a day, but to the average computer-thumping nine-to-fiver it was all wrong. The lunch-time walk to the Mexican Cantina was not enough to burn those extra calories off from breakfast. And from what I could tell by the long dinnertime lines at local restaurants, nobody was cutting back for supper either. I was beginning to see it all in a new light. The wholesale clubs, the fast food industry, the misleading labels on products, and the entire diet industry—it all had an impact on me.

The dawn of the "Wholesale Club" seemed to take people's shopping habits to a new level. Membership shopping outlets like BJ's, Costco and Sam's were giving ordinary Americans the chance to stock their pantries, shelves, refrigerators and spare rooms as if they themselves were restaurant owners. Portion sizes ran from extra large to gargantuan. Did anyone really need a 36 count of Crunch & Munch caramel popcorn or bags of pistachios the size of welcome mats? Shopping at these places and stocking up on oversized products had become a suburban tradition by the 1990s.

The fast food restaurants seemed to be on a mission to super-size the country with their sugary, salty, high-fat, high-calorie, high-carbohydrate meals, and they were succeeding by selling billions of dollars worth of food, all of which was ridiculously wrong for what the human body needed. The more I tuned into it, the more I noticed that fast food outlets had become the drug pushers of the restaurant industry. *I'll have a McSpeedball and a cocaine daiquiri to go, please.* Just to assure the public they weren't completely evil, salads were added to the menus as a consolation prize.

Some other fast food chains were merging, creating a junk food double-threat to an already sedentary pubic. Dunkin' Donuts and Baskin Robbins Ice Creams merged and suddenly appeared on the same drive-thru menus. Talk about two great tastes that taste great together. A scoop of chocolate chip ice cream in your French Vanilla coffee? Half of the population wouldn't bat an eye. Dunkin' Donuts was also offering high-fat, mucho-calorie sugar overdoses such as the "Coffee Coolatta." The nutritional impact, which was not listed on the package, amounted to essentially drinking a hot fudge sundae thru a straw. Could coffee colonics be far away?

Americans, overweight or not, were not giving their bodies what they truly needed. Other restaurants claimed to offer "healthier" options. Some chains offered items such as "Crazy Harry's Cobb Salad," an extra large salad with shredded cheese, diced hard-boiled eggs, grilled turkey, olives, bacon bits and blue cheese, all served right in its very own deep fried tortilla shell. Salad in an extra large taco shell deep-fried in oil and fat. Something told me Harry was not only Crazy, he was also dead from clogged arteries. Folks in all corners of the restaurant were ordering these types of "healthy" salads as if they were going out of style.

The madness was not limited to the fast food chains, either. The private, family-owned restaurants were upping the ante as well. In Sanibel, Florida, for instance, Julie and I were having lunch one day when I noticed the coleslaw I was eating was a little extra sweet and crunchy. I took another bite in an attempt to figure out the ingredients when I bit into an actual chunk of sugar cane! When I summoned the waiter over and inquired about the sweet taste, he responded with a sheepish grin. "Our cook has a special ingredient he puts in the coleslaw," he said. "Sugar." *Sugar?* I thought. I don't even want to know why the chicken breast I was eating was also extra sweet. I looked around the packed restaurant and saw nothing but patrons thoroughly enjoying and loving the food. They were not alone.

On television, food had it's own network and millions were tuning in daily to watch a chef named Emeril whip studio audiences into a caloric frenzy by crafting amazing high-fat high-carb recipes. People in the crowd were actually oohing, ahhing and applauding as Emeril added ingredients like garlic butter and heavy cream to his gourmet dishes. Even Emeril himself seemed to be taken aback by it all. Heck, even I was a bit taken aback by it all. My brother Rich put it all into perspective when he theorized, "The Food Network is like soft porn for the obese."

By 2003, 65% of the country was overweight, myself included. And who was to blame for all of this? Was it the Industrial Revolution? McDonald's owner Ray Kroc, responsible for such healthy alternatives as the Filet-O-Fish? Maybe not, but cooking French fries in beef lard and lying about it had to be part of the problem. Or maybe it was the cook at Graceland, who was serving Elvis fried peanut butter and banana sandwiches. Okay, maybe I'm taking this too far, but something had gone terribly wrong and it didn't stop with the folks I just mentioned.

Across town, the diet and weight loss industry continued to peddle seriously flawed approaches to people's declining health. There's no business like the snow job business, and the diet scammers were raking in over 40 billion dollars annually. For years, companies had been peddling diet pills, herbal shakes, hypnosis tapes, pre-packaged foods and "miracle" solutions, all with the pathetic slogan, "The only thing you have to lose is the weight." As if people's hard-earned money wasn't at stake. As if damaging people's metabolisms didn't mean anything. As if setting people up to fail didn't kill their self esteem, causing them to eat even more. The slickly-produced infomercials just kept coming, all featuring those powerful before and after photos that sent folks running for their credit cards. Of course if you had time to read the small print, it stated that the before and after photos were not necessarily the same two people. Diets that seemed to defy all logic were still popping up out of nowhere. Weight loss miracles such as "The Decadent Diet," where chocolate-loving fat people could enjoy vitamin-enriched candies right out of a typical container of assorted chocolates and still lose weight. There's the big guy in the infomercial with cream filling on his shirt, supposedly losing weight. If only there was room on our *List Of Obesity Felonies* for these guys.

Unfortunately, the deceptions did not stop with the flawed weight loss products.

I began to realize that the "lite," "low-cal," "low-carb," "low sugar" and "fat-free" industry was also somewhat misleading people, and I was one of them. Perhaps that was why, up to that point, I was still unable to lose the bulk of my excess weight. From the time I began my crusade, I was doing what we'd been conditioned to do. I was replacing sugar with Equal or Sweet & Low, ice cream with low-fat yogurt, salad dressing with "lite" dressing, and junk cereals with "healthy" cereals. The more I began to study ingredients, the more it dawned on me that it was more advertising than concern about health. Sure, these products were better for people, but still way off from what we truly needed to eat healthy. If a salad dressing was advertised as "low calorie," the sodium might be through the roof. If a cereal was promoted as "high in fiber and whole grain," the sugars were usually over the top. "Lite" yogurt wasn't all that light if you looked at the sugars and calories. Even the healthiest ones sold in the dairy aisle of your local supermarket needed to be policed on portion sizes. Products that were advertised as "fat-free" were not exactly free of fat. Loose label laws were allowing manufacturers a loophole to advertise that way as long as their products contained less than 1 gram of fat in a single serving. The problem was that eating five "fat-free" cookies when the serving size was one could add up to 4 grams of fat. If you checked out the carbohydrate levels on many products, they too were high as well. Almost all of the lite and low-cal products were misleading people on the portion sizes. If you read the ingredient breakdown on the side of the containers, one third of a cup equaled this many calories. One-sixteenth of a bottle contained that many calories. Exactly how healthy could a bottle of "Lite" Caesar salad dressing be at 110 calories per tablespoon? And would someone please tell me who was using "approximately two tablespoons" of it on their salads? It seemed to me that if you looked at the numbers according to what normal portion sizes were, they simply were not all that low in anything. Lower maybe, but from a weight loss perspective it was a stretch. A real eye opener. One cup of Wheaties cereal in the morning was approximately 100 calories. Grape Nuts, which promoted itself as healthy, was approximately 200 calories for one-half a cup. Again, is anybody actually sitting down for a half a cup of Grape Nuts? Well, if you're me, you're having at least 2 cups with milk and a sliced banana, and you're looking at 900 calories out of your total allotment of 1600 already consumed by 8:00 a.m.

Jaded yet? It gets better. Many products were advertising themselves as "Natural" right on the labels. Unfortunately, the FDA had never formally given the term any guidelines, rendering it useless. "Natural" meant essentially nothing, yet Americans were dropping products labeled "natural" in their shopping carts without knowledge of the unnatural processing they'd been through. Even meats such as ground sirloin, which were advertised as "lean," weren't exactly that. In fact, a three-ounce hamburger could contain as much as 15 grams of fat. On a good day

I was having six to eight ounces and was becoming baffled as to why the scale was not moving for weeks at a time.

The more I studied it, the more I agreed with the experts. A massive public health campaign—the kind that had exposed the tobacco industry—was the only chance for millions of Americans to finally face themselves, get educated and take responsibility for their weight.

On a personal level, what I learned convinced me I'd been carving out a nice maintenance plan at best for the past year and a half. Yes, there was progress, but hardly the type I needed to achieve my weight loss of 150 pounds or better. So once again, I further dissected what I was putting into my body and accepted the fact that for me, it was still too much. At times I'd get angry that I had to deny myself all the foods that I loved, but during my long walks I worked hard to accept it. Eating like that was okay for other folks, but for me, if I wanted to achieve health and happiness in my lifetime, I'd have to take things down from 10,000 cheeseburgers in paradise to one every once and a while. My body simply did not require the portion sizes of the foods I was consuming.

In the process of educating myself as to how I became fat in the first place, I also began researching the possible reasons why my current weight loss was painfully slow, and at times, nonexistent, this despite a major turnaround. In one book I read about something called *lowered resting metabolic* rate. The basic concept was that years of yo-yo dieting (I call it the 1980s) and the constant adding and sub-tracting of fat from my body may have permanently damaged my metabolism, making weight loss difficult or nearly impossible. Frightening concept. The weight loss didn't fit the work. Many people across the country were experiencing this. The frustration and mental anguish over doing the right thing with no results was extremely damaging. I thought back to my mother, whom I'd never observed overeating a day in her entire life, yet she had a weight problem. Could I have fallen into the same predicament? If I had lowered my metabolic rate, it was from too many years of losing weight and gaining it back. I learned that when you lose weight, you lose both fat and muscle. When you gain weight back after losing it, you only put back the fat. The result is that your body becomes less metabolically efficient than it was before, and it takes more work than ever to burn the calories you consume.

Think about it. All those failed diets over the years. All of the weight I'd lost and gained on diets such as Weight Watchers, Jenny Craig, and the Weight Loss

Clinic. Actually living weeks at a time on all those herbal drinks and liquid shakes. If only I'd seen how with each failed diet program I was damaging my body's ability to lose the weight. There was a price to pay physically, a price that had never quite dawned on me during all those early attempts to "get thin." Only now, in my thirties, was it all beginning to make sense to me.

I approached Melinda, hoping to develop a strategy for dealing with lowered resting metabolic rate, if in fact that was my problem. I wasn't about to give up and start hitting the drive-throughs, even though my eating disorder was beginning to drive me mad. I decided that in order to achieve the substantial weight loss I was seeking, I'd have to become somewhat of a purist. Egg whites or Egg Beaters where cereal (a bread) had been. Chinese rice vinegar where salad dressing had been. Soy milk anywhere lactose and milk had been. As far as meat, healthy spices or rubbed-on-seasonings where high sugar marinades had been. I decided to cut way back on my fruits, which I'd been having 3-4 per day. And water! Sweet, sweet water. It was time to overdose on it with 10-12 glasses per day. My big meal would take place at noon. In the afternoon, a handful of nuts such as almonds, soy nuts or wasabi nuts. According to Melinda, the fats in those were healthy. A salad with tuna for dinner, no later than 5:30 p.m. More water at night. As tough as it sounded, by this point I knew that time was a tool, and that I'd get used to it. It wouldn't always feel like a strict regime. I theorized that the amount of food I needed to eat everyday to *maintain* my current weight was a lot less than anyone actually thought. Therefore, the amount of foods I needed to eat to *lose* weight was also a lot less than anybody thought. Walking everyday. Workouts with Vincent and Sharon. A return to the tennis court when I felt physically ready. And just so you don't think I'd gone completely insane, I decided that I'd treat myself one day per week and feel good about it. Food was a beautiful thing. For those who could handle it, God Bless! I'd see them at the local steak joints once per week.

By the time Melinda and I began tweaking my new regimen in August, it had begun to look curiously like the very first diet Weight Watchers had put me on back in 1978. (They'd added many choices as the years went on.) Only now, maybe I was willing to accept it and look at it differently. Perhaps at long last I was even ready for it. Nearly 25 years earlier, the Weight Watchers diet taped to my refrigerator made me feel like I was denying myself. Now it simply felt healthy to me. It was feeding my body what it needed to have. I was getting older and that kind of eating could only serve me well. The word "diet" by this time had faded from the American language, but I was beginning to believe that the problem was that we viewed diets as a temporary food regimen to achieve our desired weights. If somehow folks could understand that proper diets consisting of fruits, vegetables and healthy meats were what the body needed permanently, it would all make sense. By autumn I'd hit my lowest weight in nearly a decade: 318 pounds. How empowering it felt. Just eighteen pounds away from a major goal. I knew that if I could break 300 I was truly ready to conquer my disease. Still, the pace was beginning to take a toll on my resolve and I expressed my frustrations to Melinda about the two-and-a-half years it had taken to lose 80 pounds (less than half the weight I needed to lose). She explained to me that my progress was exactly where I should want it to be. "By the two-and-a-half year point, most people have already lost and gained back 80 or 100 pounds, and they've hit the wall and stopped trying," she said. "Just the fact that you've slowly lost 80 pounds and your resolve to lose more continues to get stronger is a great place to be." Melinda was right, and a year from then, I surmised, if I kept on this steady course, things were going to be a lot bigger and better. Well, smaller and slimmer, if you were coming from where I was coming from. I began to accept and realize that it was a different game now in my thirties than it was in my teens and twenties. The days of losing four, six, or eight pounds in a week were long gone, and maybe for the better. Eating healthy wouldn't be enough. Exercise and eating healthy wouldn't be enough. I'd need to scrutinize what I ate everyday, and do more than just walking. I needed to work with a fitness trainer three days per week, walk or swim five days, de-emphasize food and carefully monitor my intake at every meal. My visits with Ruth would further dissect what I now realized as a complicated and complex disorder. My occasional visits with Bertram Zarins kept me from injuring myself and hurting my physical game, which was key to my success. None of this was revolutionary, and like most Americans, I was always looking for a quick fix. But for the first time in my life, I was beginning to rise to the challenge. The only way to lose weight and keep it off was the same way that had been around forever, a low-calorie, low-carb lifestyle, combined with lots of exercise. In my mid thirties, I was up to the challenge. That light feeling that I was slowly learning to appreciate was as attractive to me as food once had been. Analyzing all of this made me think twice about blowing it. I vowed to continue studying myself and dissecting the disorder. I promised to never turn a blind eye to food again. Bloated things were happening to good people, but now, at long last, a once hopeless food addict was beginning to find his way.

MAN ON A MISSION

With my newfound outlook, by the fall I'd begun to see some long-awaited results. The actual pounds continued to come off painfully slowly. However, as far as losing inches, toning up, and gaining physical energy, it was evident that I was winning at the losing game. I joined a fitness gym closer to my home called "The Boston Sports Club" (BSC) in Lexington, and added a new trainer to my team: Sharon Cummings. Sharon was 40ish, extremely knowledgeable, and in great shape, with a sense of humor to boot. The BSC club had it all: tennis courts, a pool, a giant Jacuzzi, cardio rooms, free weights, and spin and aerobics classes. I was still a bit self-conscious and joining a club like The BSC took a lot of courage. You didn't see a lot of *Gary Marinos* in there. But within two days, I was over it. I actually enjoyed being the club's token "big guy." Whether I was out on the floor or in the locker room, I received nothing but support from everyone with whom I came into contact. If you want to know where the compassionate people are in the country, the ones who actually get it, they are working out on the Cybex machines right there at the BSC in Lexington. In no time at all, I began feeling physically like a new person. Sharon was shrewd enough to break things up and keep our workouts fresh and varied. One day she took me to an isolated room to workout on what she called "Kaiser Machines." Up to this point, I was familiar with Kaiser only as a roll, but these weightlifting machines gave the word a whole new meaning. The Kaiser machines were designed to use air pressure in much the same way as shock absorbers. In fact, each machine actually had what looked like shock absorbers on them, resembling a time machine. You'd set the pressure and you were off. The coolest aspect of the Kaiser machines, in my mind, were the digital dials, which actually kept track of your repetitions on each machine. Even a guy with ADD as bad as mine could tell what the count was. Pretty convenient, huh?

Sharon had other surprises in store as well, like a massive squat machine she'd nicknamed "Mr. Smith." "Mrs. Fields" was still pretty much my speed at that point, and squats were not my favorite exercise to do. I'd be spaghetti legs for days after using the machine, and Sharon knew I dreaded it. "I thought about you all weekend," I'd say to Sharon.

"Really?" she'd ask.

"Oh yeah, pretty much every time it took me 15 minutes to get in and out of my car," I'd joke. But with each passing workout, whether I was with Sharon or on my own, I became more passionate about weightlifting.

The fat guy in me was slowly beginning to fade away and I began to feel a little bit more empowered each time. Health had become a way of life.

Another way of life change involved my new "purist" approach to eating. Bunless sirloin burgers on my George Forman Grill with ketchup and fat-free cheese were like prime rib to me by now. Raw almonds or yogurt were snacks I actually looked forward to. Salads with cherry tomatoes, celery, and shredded carrots even did it for me. All of this from the guy who had brought you "Killer Bread" just a decade earlier.

FROM PIZZA TO PROZAC

"Nobody told me there'd be days like these...strange days indeed."

—*John Lennon*

As September turned into October, something strange had begun happening in my life. On the way to becoming a healthy guy, anxiety—which had never been a problem with me—began to spike. Additionally, personal, business and family relationships all began shifting and changing in ways which even I couldn't have foreseen. At first I began to think that I was losing my mind. Specifically on the work front, relationships I'd enjoyed with performers, cameramen and production partners suddenly felt false to me. People I'd considered more than business associates now seemed like scorpions, putting on nice faces as long as our business dealings were slanted in their favor. Folks were eager to take my money, but less than eager about doing the work. Business associates did not respect my wishes, even when they were in dire need of my business. Perhaps our relationships had always been that way, but now, as I was emerging from my lifelong coma for the first time, I began to see things more clearly. The problem was not limited to work. Friendships and family relationships I'd enjoyed since childhood suddenly seemed selfish and one-sided. I realized that it was always me seeking them out, making plans, and being there for people when they needed it most. It dawned on me that some of my longtime friends weren't reciprocating. The more I studied these relationships, the more it began eating away at me. With my improving health, my thoughts became more lucid. The more lucid I became, the more jaded I became from watching people. Eventually, as I always had, I ended up in front of the mirror, asking myself if perhaps I was the aberration in this unraveling mess. Could the problem possibly be with everyone else instead of me? Had my relationships always been dysfunctional? What was happening to my life? With each passing day I became more and more disturbed by people's behaviors. While Julie and I were walking in the woods one Saturday, for the first time I broke down. "I think I'm losing it," I told my wife. "I feel like I need to part ways with 90 percent of the people in my life these days." As I went through the details of each individual relationship with Julie, it became obvious that my issues with these folks—some of whom had been with me forever—were legitimate. Life as I knew it could not go on the way it had. How had everything shifted? Around that time I was producing a video for Dr. Lillian Arleque, a motivational speaker and life coach who was beginning to make a name for herself. I explained my predicament to Lil. "Physically I'm getting healthier, but mentally, for some reason, I'm getting worse," I told her.

Dr. Lillian described the likely scenario to me. "You're taking control of your health, and therefore your life," she explained. "This is spilling over into every aspect of your life. Naturally you want to take control of your business, your marriage, and your relationships with people, the same way you are taking control of your health. The reality is that those were relationships developed with a different person than the one you are now. You are not the person you were five and ten years ago. You're seeing these relationships for what they really are. As lonely as it can be, you need to move on and find people who share the same qualities and beliefs you have." Lil's take on things made sense, perhaps too much sense. Now I began stressing to the max. *As if I'm not under enough pressure, now I need to cut ties with all these people in my life?* I thought. *How will I make a living? What kind of social life will I have?* All of these thoughts wreaked havoc in my brain. The sleeping giant had been awakened, and all I wanted to do was put things back the way they were.

I turned to Melinda next for advice. The more I told her, the more it made sense. "I don't see it as a bad thing you are realizing, Gary," she said, "I think it's a good sign that you are becoming a new person with a new sense of self-worth." I asked Melinda if she had seen this in other patients, and without hesitation she nodded her head knowingly. Melinda revealed stories of people who had left their marriages and quit their jobs. Folks who had walked out on lifelong relationships after realizing that they'd established bad ones due to the lack of self-worth. It all made sense to me, yet I shuddered at the thought of having to part ways with so many people around me. I had invited denial into my mind many times, and tried to convince myself that it was my fault that my relationships had become jaded.

To get further perspective, I turned once again to Ruth Schwartz, who made the consensus three for three. Ruth gave me solid advice for the days and months to come. "Slowly replace your existing relationships with new ones that work for you," she said. "It's the only way you can get your serenity back." I knew well what Ruth was talking about. My serenity had been seriously affected by all of this and I vowed to myself that when the day came that I had it back, I would protect it with everything I had. But for now, tough days lay ahead, no matter how much weight I lost or how healthy I got. A new person was emerging. With that realization, it occurred to me that yet another vicious cycle had begun in my life. Throughout the process of getting healthy and losing weight, I began seeing my relationships in a new light. With the reality that I would soon have to move on from these people, I began to severely stress out, making me want to eat. The problem was not just emotional. Melinda and I began to explore the notion that chronic stress had put my body into a survival mode. Body chemistry had possibly triggered a mechanism that kept it from losing weight. Could that have been my problem all along? No matter how much exercise I did or how impeccably I ate, my body refused to lose substantial weight. How's that for a circle of pain and frustration? The very thing I was trying to do—namely lose weight—was awakening parts of my brain which were creating stress, which in turn shut down my physical ability to lose weight. And you thought Weight Watchers was hard?

The result of parting ways with longtime friends and business associates was far-reaching. Marriage and family relationships hung in the balance as well. Never did I think that conquering my lifelong health issues could have such complications. I felt mentally exhausted and alone. Achieving an advanced stage of physical and mental health was forcing me to re-evaluate my life in every way. I remember telling Melinda, "No dietitian in 20 years ever told me that if I was in fact successful at losing the weight I'd essentially freak out." Melinda flashed a beautiful smile and answered, "That's probably correct, Gary," she said. "And why would they have told you that? Then you'd never have even tried to get healthy." I was beginning to understand it all. Eating tons of food and having a weight problem for all those years had kept me from dealing with many essential things in my life, including dealing with dysfunctional relationships. "Freaking out" wasn't such a bad thing after all, because it meant I was moving forward and getting healthy. Melinda then reiterated her earlier viewpoint. "You've turned off the food valve, Gary. You're essentially detoxing and you're freaking out. For all those years, food was your fix, and now you're changing the connection you have with it." Boy, the things they leave off of all those weight loss infomercials!

Based on all the advice I was getting, I knew it was time to pull back and re-evaluate my world. I decided that after years of being a social animal at parties, events and work get-togethers, it was time to become a bit of a recluse. My serenity was at stake, and I had to pull back for a bit to figure things out. I also vowed that I would not stay reclusive forever, just until I was ready to move on with my life. Some people lose weight to look better physically. I was completely reinventing a new life for myself. Never had I thought things would get so complicated, but the wheels were in motion and there was no turning back now.

SPIN CONTROL

"What do you say we try something different today?" my trainer Sharon shrewdly suggested in an attempt to get my mind off the numbers on the scale and back into the workout.

I asked Sharon what she had in mind. "Take a spin class with me," she responded.

"Me? A spin class? Don't you have to be in really good shape to take one of those?" I asked.

"No. Everybody thinks that's the case, but it's for everybody," she explained. I shot Sharon my best *thank you but you know you're giving me too much credit* look. "No really, this class has a fun instructor and he plays great music. You'll do great," she said. As much as I appreciated Sharon's faith in me, I'd grown a bit skeptical over the course of the last year of these fitness-trainer-types like Vincent and Sharon. I appreciated their faith that I could perform the same workouts as their thin clients and I had no doubt that they knew their stuff, but my instincts were that because they had never been overweight, they might not understand just how awkward, painful and devoid of energy a big person feels during these workouts. Now I've been on both sides of the scales and I know that an overweight person is severely handicapped, compared to an out-of-shape normal-sized person. You just don't hit the mats with the same energy or stamina.

I asked Sharon one last time if she really thought I was ready for a spin class.

"I don't know, Hon, are you really sure I don't have to be in better shape for something like this?" I asked, looking for any excuse to bag out, just as I'd been doing my entire life.

Sharon responded with her usual confidence and sweet style. "No, don't be ridiculous, there are all sizes and shaped people in there." After a few more minutes of this type of *should I, shouldn't I?* bantering, I caved and agreed to the spin class. The healthier I became, the more I was willing to try new things anyway.

Okay, first problem right out of the gate. Sharon and I walked into the workout room, picked out our bikes and look around. There wasn't one person in the room who looked like me. There were about 30 people, young and old, and everybody seemed to be in phenomenal shape. They all seemed spin-savvy and familiar with each other. Right off the bat I was in my trademark *why did I ever agree to do this?* mode. Now at this point, I hadn't been on any kind of a bicycle for well over fifteen years, and when I hopped on it, the former fat guy in me immediately looked around for the TV mount and the hors d'oeuvres tray extension. "The instructor won't be here for another ten minutes, but you'll want to jump on and warm up," said Sharon.

What I want to do is warm up a chicken parm sandwich, I thought as I jumped on the bike. At this point, despite the 75-pound weight loss, there was still plenty of *which way to the nearest drive-thru* in me, and my confidence lagged in situations like this. Second problem. After pedaling the bike for ten minutes, I was ready to take a break, but an announcement was made that the instructor was running behind and would be another 15 minutes. I looked around to see if anybody was going dismount and grab a granola bar somewhere. No such luck. Everybody continued pedaling and conversing with each other. By the time the instructor showed up and slipped Lenny Kravitz' "American Woman" into the CD player, the warm-up phase had already exhausted me and taken me down for the count. Third problem. The guy instructing the class was an animal. A serious "no pain, no gain" type kid, all of 24 years old with a massive, sculptured build, and a solid set of vocal chords. I found myself wondering if the "Bulldog" from my childhood football days had had a son.

"All right, people, let's hit it!" he shouted. I could feel the dread oozing throughout my mind and body with that sinking *this is gonna be bad* feeling.

In the mirror in front of me I had a bird's eye view of what the rest of the class was doing. Rather than getting busted for aggravated mopery in the spin class, I just mimicked them for a bit. "Everybody down, resistance of four!" yelled Bulldog Jr. *Resistance of what?* I thought, as I hunkered down on the bike, closely watching everyone in the mirror. *What the hell is resistance?* I wished I'd resisted Sharon when she suggested this idea, but now I was in the class and the experience had become a runaway train. "Okay, everybody take your resistance down to three and speed it up!" bawled the instructor. I looked around. Everybody was pedaling as fast as they could. It occurred to me at that point that if I could see everybody in the mirror, they could also see me. Of course most people would have figured that out right at the beginning. I jammed on the pedals and brought the speed to a much faster level, but the instructor continued his yelling, wanting more, more and more. "Resistance of six, Go! Go! Go!" he bellowed. *Excuse me,* I thought, *did you learn this screaming routine from your dad?*

Just when my body hit the breaking point, a new song with a super fast beat came on and the instructor called for a new addition to the process. On his count, the girls and guys switched off and pedaled their bikes as fast as humanly possible for a certain period of time. When the women fast pedaled, the men pedaled at a slow warm-up pace and cheered the girls on as loudly as possible. When the men were up, the women would do the same, providing moral support and team spirit. Only one problem: there were all of 3 guys in the entire room and about 27 girls. *Just what I need,* I remember thinking, *more attention!*

"All right, ladies, on five, four, three, two, one!" And there was Sharon next to me, hunched down on her bike, pedaling at lightning speed.

"Yeah, Sharon!" the other guys and I cheered her on. The girl was in shape, that much was for sure. I actually enjoyed cheering Sharon on so much, I forgot that my turn was coming. A second later I heard those fateful words.

"Okay, guys, get ready in five, four, three, two, one!" By then I was in outright survival mode, just looking to play along and not cause too much of a scene. At this point I reluctantly got the entire room's undivided attention. I put my best game face on and began jamming on the pedals like there was no tomorrow. "Nice! Go, Gary!" yelled Sharon. I closed my eyes and waited for the instructor's voice.

"Okay, slow down, guys; nice work. Ladies, in five, four, three, two, one! I made it, and seemingly without incident. As I cheered the women on, I began to feel more confident *Hey, I'm actually doing it. I'm actually doing all right.* Isn't it funny how in life, just when you're about to get a little cocky, you realize you're a complete buffoon?

Back to the spin class. We switched between guys and girls a couple of times by then, and our turn was coming up. "Guys, resistance of five in five, four, three, two, one! Once again I hunkered down on the bike and pedaled as fast as I could, with the eyes of the entire class on the two other guys and me, but this time when I studied the situation in the mirror I noticed something significant. The other guys were pedaling a lot more slowly than I was and seemed to be struggling even more. For a brief second I wondered whether I was, in fact, in great shape after all for a man of size. A second later it occurred to me what all this resistance stuff the instructor was talking about was. In the middle of the bike, between everybody's legs, was a dial with the word, you guessed it, "Resistance." Here I was thinking I was a hero and my resistance dial, the one that makes it harder to pedal, has never left zero. Knowing I could never keep up with the class of fit, buff and seasoned spin people, I decided to do a little spin control of my own. I decided I'd do the best acting job I'd ever turned in. I put my best fake game face on and gave the resistance dial a phony quarter turn to the right. As the instructor continued yelling to the guys to alternate their bike's resistance between two and eight, I simply watched the speed of the other bikers in the mirror and followed along with what they were doing. They sped up, I'd speed up. They adjusted their resistance, I'd act like I was adjusting it too. They had pained looks on their faces, and I'd turn on my best Rocky Balboa expression. The girl/guy alternating routine seemed to go on forever, and I was getting pretty good at the game. Even with all those fake adjustments I was making on the resistance dial, it occurred to me that I was still getting a pretty good workout.

The next exercise was a doozy. But any good workout, even a fake one, ups the ante as it goes along, right? This time the instructor had us do what essentially amounted to aerobics, but on a bike. I was already aerodynamically challenged and this was where my acting job began to come apart at the seams. If the resistance was left at zero, but it was actually supposed to be on six (keep in mind we're talking about opposite ends of the spectrum here), it's tough to pedal slowly enough to look legit. Once you're pedaling fast enough—with no resistance—the pedals actually have a mind of their own and take you for the run of your life. Get the visual? I was trying to act like I was struggling to pedal, and about the only thing I was struggling with was to get the damn pedals to slow down and stop spinning so fast so it looked like my resistance was actually turned on. Right around that time, I decided I'd had enough. I'd been on the bike pedaling for better or for farce—er, for worse—for the better part of an hour. I slipped off the bike, motioned to Sharon, giving her a thank you wink, and headed for my favorite part of the workout: the heated Jacuzzi.

Back in the locker room after a hot, extra long shower, I ran into one of the older participants from the spin class. He was a very nice 60-something guy named

Murray or Sammy or something. "Hey, nice job today," he said with a smile. "You didn't know it, but I was watching you in the mirror during the spinning class". *That's funny,* I thought, *I was watching you too, as in every move you made.* "You kept up with the rest of us very well," he continued.

"Thanks," I responded, embarrassed over my zero-resistance acting job.

"You know," he continued, "we've all been together for about seven years in that class, and you kept up like one of the team." Now that caught my attention.

"Together as a team? Did you say seven years?" I queried.

"Yep. All of us have been taking that same spinning class for 7 or 8 years, and this instructor is the hardest yet." Now the fact that there weren't any folks like me in the class made sense. I saw now why everybody seemed to know what they were doing on the bikes, and how they always seemed familiar with the instructor's spinning routines. I felt a little betrayed until I remembered that it was a decent workout, combined with a stellar acting job.

"You're in pretty good shape for a big guy. Keep up the good work," he said, the smile still planted on his face. I threw my gym bag around my shoulder and headed for the door. "Thanks," I responded. *I'd like to thank the Academy...*

DOLCE VITA
(The Sweet Life)

Around the middle of November, 2002, a holiday party invitation arrived from my clients Ellen Burnett and Linda Simon. The two savvy and successful women owned an event-planning company in the area called "Best Of Boston" and I'd been doing business with them for a couple of years. A wonderful client inviting me to their year-end holiday party sounded like fun. The trouble was that the party was at none other than Dolce Vita, one of my favorite Italian restaurants of all time. Dolce Vita was located in Boston's North End. Although it hadn't made my *Top Five List Of Perverse Places,* it was definitely in my Top Ten. The restaurant was owned and operated by a man named Franco, a jovial man with a permanent smile only partially hidden beneath his long, grey mustache. Franco was one of the few men I'd let kiss me on both cheeks in public, and not just because he'd greet me warmly at the door and serenade me with his guitar playing. His restaurant served up serious Italian dishes such as Fettuccine Bolognese and Pollo alla Marsala, not to mention metabolism-jarring desserts. When Julie and I received the E-vite, I vowed to be impeccable in the two weeks leading up to the party because I knew I'd be putty in Franco's hands the moment I walked in the door and smelled the food. The "All or Nothing" syndrome might have been defeated, but a former food addict still needs to treat himself now and then, right?

I picked up the phone and scheduled two sessions with Sharon, my trainer at The Boston Sports Club in Lexington—one for the current week and one for the day of the party at Dolce Vita. "That way," I told Julie, "I'll walk in there feeling all right about treating myself."

Week one went fantastic. Healthy meals and snacks, with Sharon guiding me through my usual rounds of cardio, weight training and workouts on the mats. By the end of week one I already felt I'd made some serious progress. You know the feeling you get when you've hit the gym everyday, kept it to 1600 calories, and even hit the bed before 11 p.m. at night? I was feeling terrific and extremely curious to jump on the scale and physically see if I'd lost any weight. Put your seat in it's upright position and strap yourself in, because now the fun starts.

In the men's locker room after my usual round of pool laps I noticed a good old-fashioned scale. Not a digital one, not a fancy high-tech one, just a good old-fashioned slider scale that had always given me the real deal without the second-guessing. I jumped on the scale with visions of an impressive weight loss paving the way for an even more impressive Dolce Vita outing. On the scale I fixed the large slider to the usual 300-pound setting, and the little one towards the 20-pound mark. Immediately the scale pointed down, meaning my settings were wrong. "Could I possibly be under 300 pounds?" I asked myself. Considering that I'd weighed in at 321 with Melinda just a week before, it just didn't seem possible. When I adjusted the big setting to 250 and the little one to 35 pounds, the scale seemed to level off, revealing a weight of 285 pounds. *Huh?* I thought. *No way. I've been good. Not that good.* I immediately stepped off the scale, reset every thing to zero and stepped back up to try again. Incredibly, the scale read 285 pounds again. Now those kinds of numbers were music to my ears, but before getting too elated I took a reality check. *Forty pounds in a week? I don't think so. Are my clothes forty pounds looser? No way.* That *I'd notice.* I studied the scale, looking for broken parts, chewing gum stuck in all the wrong places, perhaps a sign that read "out of order." I became perplexed and baffled. To my knowledge, these scales had always given solid readings. That's why most professionals used them, right? Now I was looking at the possibility of being under 300 pounds for the first time in a decade and not sure if I should be celebrating or not. I weighed myself another time. Okay, maybe 3 or 4 times (the numbers were in the right direction, after all) and then headed for my locker to get changed. While I was tying my sneakers, a good-looking young guy with a fit and well-sculptured body walked up and jumped on the scale. I watched his face for any sign of bewilderment. Nothing. Would he jump off and try again? Surely his reading had to be 30 to 40 pounds off if mine was. Nothing. He jumped off and headed for the showers. I was confused. I jumped on after he left and came up with the same 285 pound reading. The next day when I arrived at the gym I noticed another guy, this one with a huge build and thin waist, on the scale, looking at his reading. "Excuse me, but that scale is a little off, isn't it?" I asked.

The guy looked at me and then back at the scale expressionless. "Not really," he answered as he jumped off. Now I was even more confused. Ten seconds later another man, this one in his late 40s, stepped on. Alarmingly, I moved toward the area where the scale was.

"Hey, that thing is toast, isn't it?" I asked.

The man looked at me sarcastically, and said, "Oh yeah, it's definitely toast all right." I recognized the look. It was the old *the Big Guy is in some serious denial* look.

"No, no," I said, lightening up a bit. "I like the numbers, I just think it's off a bit."

"Maybe a little," said the man, becoming more serious, "but it's tough for this type of scale to be that far off."

"Gotcha" I responded, sounding as if he'd told me something I already didn't know.

As the days went on, I became obsessed with the scale's accuracy, literally stalking guys in the locker room as they headed to jump on the scale. My next appointment with Melinda wasn't for another two weeks and I was desperate to see if I'd dropped some serious weight. At the gym, I'd become like George Costanza from Seinfeld, obsessing about everybody else's reading on the scale. The week of the Dolce Vita party I walked into the locker room to get changed. As soon as I put my gym bag down on the bench I noticed a 20-something guy with a full head of hair, huge build and star-quarterback smile on the scale. I recognized that a distinct look of confusion had come over his face. "Hey...hey!" I yelled, tripping over a bench as I rushed toward him, my pants halfway down to my knees. "Tell me that scale isn't toast!" He looked at me briefly and then back at the reading on the scale. "Oh, yeah. This thing is way off," he answered.

"Thank you!" I responded, vindicated by what I'd suspected all along. Then the guy dropped the bomb.

"I'm at least thirty pounds heavier on this scale than I should be," he said. My jaw dropped. "Thirty pounds heavier? You mean lighter, right?" I asked incredulously.

"Nope, heavier. I weighed myself yesterday at home," he responded, shaking his head as he headed to the sauna. Now I was really confused. I jumped on the scale again to see if perhaps I too would be thirty pounds heavier for some reason. You do the math. I was 321 last time I weighed in. I had a great two weeks, so perhaps I was now down to 318 pounds. If the scale gave him a reading 30 pounds above what he weighed, my number should read somewhere around 348, correct? Well, one man's 30 pound weight gain is another man's loss, I guess. Completely mystified, I jumped on the scale yet again. The scale still read 285 pounds.

"Oh-My-God! Now this has gotten ridiculous." I quipped. "The best two weeks of my life and I've got the Bermuda Triangle of scales here."

The next day as Sharon and I lay on the mats, stretching before our workout, she noticed that I was perplexed and detached. I shared with her my dilemma over the mystery scale.

"Wow, that is strange!" Sharon said with a humorous tone. I guess it was pretty funny. A big guy obsessing about a scale that apparently is right out of the Twilight Zone.

"Hey, is that Rod Serling over on the Stairmaster?" I joked, just to let her know I hadn't completely lost my mind.

"Actually, I heard they removed the scale to have the calibration adjusted, so don't worry too much about what the numbers are," Sharon said, solving the mystery.

◆   ◆   ◆

"What do you say we try something different today?" Sharon shrewdly suggested in an attempt to get my mind off the numbers on the scale and back into workout mode. A little déjà vu had begun to settle in at that point.

"The last time you said those words I ended up over my head in a spin class full of seven-year veterans," I said to Sharon as she laughed. I liked Sharon's approach: keep it fresh and new. My other trainer Vincent had stressed the importance of that earlier, but I politely declined whatever she had in mind. With the Dolce Vita Party just two days away, I wanted to do something I knew would burn some calories.

"I think I'll hit the pool and swim some laps," I said. At the pool I hit the water hard. Backstroke down. Breast stroke up. Free style back. Side stroke. Under water stroke. Here a stroke, there a stroke, everywhere a stroke stroke.

◆   ◆   ◆

Okay, December 7, 2002. D-Day—or Dolce Vita Day. My butt was still in pain from the spin class. I still had no idea what I weighed because the Bermuda Triangle Scale had apparently been taken to be fixed somewhere. As I wrapped up a late afternoon workout at the gym, visions of gourmet Italian dishes filled my head. Like a kid on Christmas Eve, I strategized over which gift I'd open first. *I'll hit the Lobster Ravioli first, then move right on to the Pollo al Forno Chicken, topped with prosciutto and mozzarella cheese. Yeah, that's the ticket. Then I'll do some damage to the grilled vegetable antipasto, but save room if there's Scaloppini Boscaiola.* Always the addict. By the time I got to my car in the parking lot it had been snowing for a couple of hours, and for a brief moment I considered calling Julie and canceling. I'd made plans to meet her in the city to attend the party together. I'd worked so hard that week to be able to make a mess of myself at Dolce Vita, and as any food lover knows, once we've made up our minds we're going to treat ourselves, there's no turning back. We want to be *naughty*, correct? So I placed myself right smack in the middle of the epidemic known as rush hour traffic for the wrong reason. *Food!* It took nearly an hour and a half to travel the seven miles from the gym in Lexington, down Route 128 to the Massachusetts Turnpike. From there I went against the commute and slipped into town fairly easily. Now in Massachusetts these days we have five seasons: winter, spring, summer, fall and road construction. And in Boston we had the mother of all construction projects—the $14 billion dollar Big Dig. When I hit the Big Dig traffic I exasperatingly phoned Julie on her cell phone. By now we were a full two hours late for the Best Of Boston party, and the snow continued to fall. "What do you think, should we can it?" asked Julie.

"No. Absolutely not. For two reasons. First I RSVP'd that we'd be attending, and second the chow, and not necessarily in that order," I responded. Okay, cut to the North End a full 30 minutes later. I'd parked my car a mile away in an $18.00 lot, not even noticing that the fine folks from the Best Of Boston were offering free valet parking right in front of the restaurant. That's what happens when you're a man with ADD on a mission to eat. The party had begun at 5:00

p.m. It was now close to 8:00 p.m. I met Julie, and when we walked in I made the rounds, greeting agents, clients and competitors alike, all of this with my eye on the sides of the room where the buffet was set up. By the time I made it over, another 20 minutes had slipped away and the once heaven-sent buffet was seriously depleted. The party was winding down and the waiters were moving half-empty platters to make room for the dessert. Julie and I filled our plates and sat down as quickly as possible. Now you can't talk business with people while jamming food in your mouth. Of course when we sat down, we found ourselves at a table of inquisitive talkers. "What does your company do?" and "How can we do more business next year?" types. In reality, we ate very little. Julie tried to convince me that all my hard work had not been in vain.

"Look at it this way; you can continue this healthy period without falling off," she offered. Now Hell hath no fury like a dieter looking to treat himself, right? We feel gypped. We want to even the score, so after all of 40 minutes at the party Julie and I put our coats on, thanked our gracious hosts and headed for the car. It was still snowing and I was still looking to settle the score. "Let's head over to Mike's Pastry to grab a cannoli," I said to Julie. For those of you not familiar with this legendary slice of heaven, feel free to leaf back to the Top Five Perverse Places, as Mike also owned a landmark pastry and coffee place as famous for its cannoli as Boston was for its baked beans. "No. That's ridiculous!" said Julie as I grabbed her hand and headed across the street to Mike's.

"Don't argue with me," I said. "I came to eat and I'm not leaving till I do!" Not exactly your average lover's quarrel, is it? The girl was a saint. As usual, the place was packed with people drinking coffee and in line to buy pastry. I asked Julie if she wanted to join me in a chocolate-covered, cream-filled, chocolate chip cannoli.

"No, I don't want anything," she answered in an annoyed, yet supportive tone. Acting as if I hadn't hear her, I ordered two cannolis anyway, figuring she'd pass once again, forcing me to eat both. Modern day food addicts like me will always publicly deny making moves like this, but trust me, we all do it. I paid for the cannoli and tried to convince Julie to sit down at a table and eat them immediately, but by this time she was annoyed by the whole scene. By the time we trudged our way back to the parking lot where the car was, Julie was looking to blow off some steam. "I'll scrape the snow off the car," she said.

"Okay," I responded enthusiastically. I put the radio on, turned the heat up, put the driver's seat into recline position and proceeded to eat both cannolis. There's a real Norman Rockwell for you. Right, folks? Call this one "Scenes From An Addict." There's the freezing wife in the snowstorm scraping the window and peering in with agitation while the husband is in the warm car listening to Jimmy Buffett's "Cheeseburger In Paradise," while he eats cannolis with a big stupid smile on his face. Cigarette, anyone?

By late December I was doing the usual year-end shuffle, producing the final projects and live shows with Harmon-Marino and hitting the gym about every other day. On a business basis, 2002 was strong, considering that most of my clients were on the verge of extinction in the midst of the shattered economy. Our jobs had run the gamut Comedy shows with meat loaf dinners one night, and Meat Loaf himself the next night. Even at work, the food references never seemed to stop.

As the year lumbered along to a close, I became melancholy and perplexed at the realization that my health goals would never be met in 2002. Now 24 pounds is 24 pounds, but after two-and-a-half years, I had still only lost about a third of the weight I needed to lose.

Perhaps it was the scene in the car with the cannolis, or maybe it was the fact that the scale hadn't moved in six months, but I began to wonder if I'd ever honestly achieve true health. Despite a strong finish to the year with healthy meals and marathon workouts, my weight still hung around the 318-320 mark, and for a brief moment, I began to feel lost all over again. It had been over two years since I'd started. I'd spent countless hours with nutritionists, trainers, therapists and well-meaning supporters. I'd studied nutrition and self-improvement articles, tweaked recipes and defeated the dreaded "All or Nothing" syndrome. I'd designed a non-profit foundation to fight obesity, begun work on a unique weight loss walk and a personal journey/self-help book. I'd logged over 1,300 miles walking and had rid myself the trappings of an office and employees. Yet despite this monumental effort, I was still a severely overweight individual. Depressed, I unloaded all of this on the same person I'd always unloaded on: my therapist Ruth Schwartz. How or why Ruth listened to people talk about their frustrations all day was an increasing mystery to me. I honestly began to feel bad, constantly venting my feelings at her. Could anyone actually get any satisfaction out of this as a career? The success rates for weight loss were so pathetic and poor. Could she really continue to listen to folks like me go on and on about how bad it sucked? Apparently the answer was yes. That Ruth was one sweet and calming woman all right, who in no time had me feeling like a new man. "You have to take stock of your progress, Gary, and keep in mind that the overall goal here is *health* in general, not just weight loss," she said. "Remember that it's about the big picture. Do not lose sight of the fact that you are a healthier person than when you started." When I thought about it, Ruth had a point. My 80-pound weight loss had not only occurred, but had been kept off. My Sleep Apnea problem seemed to have drifted away with only one third of the weight gone. My mind and ability to think was clearer. Most days I felt energetic and ready to rise to the challenges that life and work always seemed ready to throw at me. At the gym, my trainers were constantly assuring me that I was in great shape, despite my still-lingering weight problem.

"You hit these workouts with the same speed, stamina and repetitions as my thin clients," was one trainer's comment. Once I tuned in to it, I noticed that my breathing was better. I could (and would) run four flights of stairs and not even breathe heavy or feel any pain in my legs. My eating was 100 percent healthier than it was in 2000, and I actually enjoyed the right foods. My resting heart rate had gone from 90 to 81, which suggested that my heart was much healthier than it had been in 2000. Tests revealed that even my blood had become healthier, thanks to all of the eating right and exercising. My HDL (the good cholesterol) had gone from 49 to 56. My LDL (bad cholesterol) from 122 to 104. Total cholesterol went from 189 to 171, and my blood pressure from 130 over 60 to 106 over 80. Finally, my body mass index had gone from 62 to 46.6. I'd learned tons of facts about nutrition, exercise and human behavior. As for my clothes, I'd gone down several sizes and was back into clothes I'd bought around the time of my wedding in 1993.

I came to realize through my Dream Team that the process of constantly taking stock of your progress was of vital importance, especially in a weight loss situation which affects your body slowly over time. By taking stock in a positive way, it motivated me and gave me the resolve I needed to push further.

At each meeting with Ruth or Melinda in which I expressed my frustrations, I was encouraged to accept my struggle for the disease it was. Acceptance was important. It is, for good reason, the basis today for every Overeaters Anonymous and Alcoholics Anonymous 12-step program out there. Acceptance would help pave the way in my universe for a true healing. Too deep here? Let me spell it out. I came to believe that this disease was given to me for a reason: it was my challenge in life to beat. Ruth always encouraged me to look at the big picture. It went beyond a simple diet plan or set of workout rules. It was more than counting calories and eating less. Perhaps it was a challenge I had been ignoring for the better part of my life. I began to theorize that it was what I was put here to conquer. Now I was in the midst of tackling it. On the other side of the struggle, if I were able to overcome the odds and beat it I'd be truly a happier, healthier, more developed and evolved person.

The acceptance part was key. From my friend and client Tom Hayes I'd learned about something called the "The Law Of Acceptance," or accepting the good and bad sides of everything that happened in life. The decisions I'd made and the things I'd prayed for came within both sides of the positive/negative spectrum. I needed to be at peace with that. In the process of accepting what had happened in my life, I would also have to take responsibility for my actions. If you've been reading this, you all know about my part in this weight problem: all those *misadventures* involving heisted dinners and manipulation involving food. My disease wasn't to blame for that; I was. This behavior had, in fact, contributed to the bloated and lost caricature of the human I'd become for all those years. I paid the price dearly for it. In the end, life is a test of acceptance and forgiveness. In my heart I needed to forgive myself for my actions in all those situations when there was no one else in the room but me. I needed to forgive the higher power who created me for putting this challenge upon me. If I could forgive Him for the challenge I'd been given and accept the outcome of my health struggle, for better or worse, then perhaps what I'd been working so hard for over the past two years could actually happen. The fact was that my life and relationships would change dramatically if I became a fit and healthy person. I needed to accept both the positives and the negatives that would come with those changes and not be angry with God. I'd already spent half my lifetime being angry at Him. I needed to be at peace with the both the good and the bad of everything I asked for in life. Now it was time to change in mind and soul so I could at last change physically. Deep in my heart, even during my younger years, I'd always known it would take a monumental mental and spiritual awaking to get this powerful disease under control—an epiphany, followed by a cleansing that would lead me to a new 'GO' point in life. I may have only lost 24 pounds in 2002, but at long last I'd learned how to do it. I'd learned what I needed to do to truly lose all those extra pounds and stay healthy. I'd discovered the value of the "Long Term Fix" versus the "Short Term Fix." No, I wouldn't be a male model anytime soon, but I'd probably live to see my grandkids. The past two and a half years had been an invaluable education and training. Now I finally felt ready to do what needed to be done. More importantly, at last I had found a set of beliefs I could accept. When a man establishes a belief system that he can live by, he is reborn. At 37 years of age I'd at long last discovered that set of beliefs. As 2003 loomed, I viewed it with an optimism and inner peace I'd never experienced before. A true second chance at the journey. Life could be sweet again...*Dolce Vita*.

TRIPLE THREAT '03

The Whydah was an English pirate treasure ship lost off the coast of Cape Cod during the great storm of 1717. The brutal storm that sank the ship not only claimed the lives of all aboard, but it also sent the only documented collection of pirate treasure to the bottom of the ocean for over 250 years. Captain Barry Clifford spent years trying to pinpoint the location of the sunken wreck after growing up hearing stories about The Whydah from his Uncle Bill. Even though most onlookers were skeptical that the wreck had ever existed, Barry Clifford pushed on with a tenacity and admirable determination that seemed to defy all odds. In 1983, Clifford was tantalizingly close to silencing his critics and finding the Whydah, when his Uncle Bill became very ill. He carried on with his search and about one year before his historical discovery of the wreck in 1984, he visited his uncle one last time in the hospital on his deathbed. Although his uncle never lived to see the actual finding of the ship, he could tell from the gleam in his nephew's eye that he was about to find it. Indeed, Clifford had narrowed the location of the pirate treasure ship to an undeniable strip of ocean about 1500 yards off the coast of Eastham, MA (which is today known as Wellfleet).

In the winter of 2003 I had that very same gleam in my eyes that Barry Clifford had had when he knew he had located the lost treasures of the Whydah. In fact, by February, I'd become a triple threat.

The experiences of learning and dissecting the last two years seemed to permeate my mind, and suddenly my lifelong food addiction seemed to lose it's hold over my life. Elvis had left the building and my addiction had left my body.

I hadn't discovered buried treasure, but I'd certainly found a treasure trove of knowledge on how to become a healthy person, and I'd found a new confidence and attitude, the likes of which I'd never had before. I felt empowered. I felt strong. Health-wise, I was simply on fire. For the first time since I was a kid, I had finally gained control over my food issues and was enjoying a lifestyle of healthy eating and exercising. I'd learned portion sizes, calorie counting and how to see through the deceptive advertising. Most importantly, I was happy with 1600 calories of low carbohydrate, healthy food every day.

At the gym, my intensive workouts suddenly went from decaf to speedball. If my trainer wanted 16 reps, I would give her 20. Between free weights or Cybex machines, while Sharon adjusted machines for seat settings and weights, I'd circle the area with brisk walks or light jogs. God forbid I let my heart rate go down, right? I'd hit the gym, pumped and ready to feel "the burn," as my fellow fitness junkies referred to it. In fact I was so into working out by 2003 that I suddenly began working out without a trainer. Now most people who work out will tell you that you always do a better workout when you are with a trainer. I happen to agree, but suddenly I was able to enter the gym alone and hit the routine pretty hard. I knew the weights, seat settings, angle adjustments, and everything else. I had accountability to myself after each set. I had the ability to honestly assess my workouts and ask myself "Now did I really hit it hard or was I in autopilot?" Most days I was hitting things hard, and more importantly, loving it.

Just to round out my *triple threat* approach and guarantee my success, I signed up for a 16-week cardiac risk and nutrition course at Salem Hospital, not far from the State College where I once ate pizza and drank beer like there was no tomorrow. My, how things had changed!

The class had been Melinda's suggestion, and it was yet another smart move on her part.

The program was further education and conditioning for me. It put me in a classroom setting and gave me a greater understanding of what had gone wrong and how to fix it. Saturated fats. Hydrated substances. I learned things I'd long been ignoring, and the more I learned the more fascinated I became. For example, did you know that pork, universally advertised as "The Other White Meat," is actually a red meat? That McDonald's, at one time deep-fried their french fries in beef lard? Or how about the fact that stretching before exercising can be hazardous to your health? Apparently cold muscles could be damaged. Who knew? The process of hydrogenation is responsible for the harmful amounts of transfats contained in margarine spreads. The class gave me the chance to push my knowledge of nutrition and exercise further than it ever had been before. It also gave me the chance to fulfill my role as the class clown one last time.

Teacher: "Does anyone know why it's important to flex our muscles after workouts?"

Me: "So we can be more flexible?"

Teacher: "Losing weight is a slow process. You've got to ask yourself how long it took to get this heavy. Gary, for instance, how long did it take you to get this way?"

Me: "Not long. Not very long at all. Pretty much from the time I set eyes on my first slice of carrot cake, it was all over for me."

The risk reduction course had helped to kick my recovery into high gear, and in April of 2003 I stepped on the scale and saw the numbers "297." I'd done it! I'd not only cracked the 300 mark, but in my heart of hearts I knew I'd kissed the 300s good-bye forever. I'd evolved. Unlike that fateful day four years earlier when the numbers had read "397," there was only one thought in my head:

"I'm back"

I'd finally managed to turn the tables on myself, and a noticeable air of victory surrounded me that spring wherever I went. Friends and co-workers took notice and congratulated me constantly. My cousin Michele's husband, Doug, greeted me with lines like, "Hey it's you! No, actually it's half of you!"

Clients would hit me with lines like, "It looks like you've learned a thing or two about losing weight, huh?" Or, "So & so said they saw you at the club the other night and didn't even recognize you." Maybe it was the gleam in my eye, or perhaps the workouts were giving me the appearance of weighing less than I did; whatever it was, 2003 was a very sweet year for me. Personally, it was a significant, victorious and magical time in my life. Well, almost magical.

As 290 became 270, I still had my moments of relapses and weight plateaus, but what was different at this point was my feelings about food. Let me give you an example. For the better part of my teens, twenties, and half of my thirties, I was the type of person who would look at a slice of raspberry cheesecake or steak calzone and say, "You complete me." It was a deep impulse and emotional experience with no negotiating. I had to have it. By early 2003, if I was at a party eating a slice of cheesecake or calzone in the corner, I'd be laughing at myself, usually with my wife by my side. I'd eat it with a smile on my face and be thinking to myself, *This is so stupid eating this. This slice has to be 1200 calories. So good, and yet it's wrong on so many levels. I can't wait to work out tonight and eat healthy tomorrow morning.* See the difference? I didn't need it. It was a weak moment in time. I'd eat the cheesecake because it was there, it was delicious looking, I was socializing, I was only human and once in a while you've got to live.

In addition to my feelings about food, my ability to get back on my healthy weight loss routine was razor sharp. My resolve was always strong, but by now it was like…well, riding a bike.

In April I flew to Los Angeles to represent Matty Blake for a talent showcase at the Hollywood Improvisation. Always rushing to get somewhere, I was one of the last to board the plane. (Hey, losing a lot of weight doesn't help you with time management!) On the jet it turned out I had a window seat, and when I joined the other two guys in my row I felt unusually comfortable. Now could the airline spare a little more room? Sure. But the point is that I sat in the window seat, unfazed. My seat belt was buckled with room to spare, and it dawned on me that I'd forgotten to ask for a seat belt extension. Apparently things had changed and none was needed. If you were on that flight, I was the guy in row 18, seat C, the one with the permanent smile planted on my face.

When it was time for the in-flight meal, I pulled my tray out in front of me, completely level with room to spare. For the first time in years, I was about to eat airplane food again. Of course one bite of the omelet reminded me that I'd been missing exactly nothing. Where the Delta Diet Plan had been all these years, I had no idea.

In Los Angeles I was on my A game, working out at the hotel gym every night and walking Wilshire and Santa Monica Boulevard every day. This was a brand new me. Never had I worked out in a hotel gym or actually lost weight on the road. But suddenly there I was, a changed man. At meetings with talent agencies and production companies I was attentive, energetic and invigorated about Harmon-Marino business again.

My new approach to life didn't stop with work, either. Vacations became a new experience altogether. In September, Julie and I took an extended vacation in Miromar Lakes, Florida, house-sitting for family friends Dave and Cheryl Slocum.

In Miromar, I learned to transition my typical *All you can eat without leaving your chaise lounge* vacation into a three-week stay at a health resort. We ate healthy, walked every day, took water aerobics classes (it's harder than it looks, trust me) and gave the word "rejuvenation" a whole new meaning. I also reintroduced the game of tennis back into my life, taking lessons and playing almost daily with Julie. Athletically speaking, I loved it. Backhand. Forehand. Running between the service line and base line with no problem. Mr. Pivot was a thing of the past. Now don't get me wrong, I might not be a great tennis player yet, but in time, who knows?

I also began buying and reading health magazines such as Men's Fitness and Men's Health. The articles made sense to me and the information I gleaned was invaluable. Intellectually, I was discovering a whole new world.

By the end of 2003 I'd hit 268 pounds and my wife was lauding the return of "the 'old Gary' face." Frankly, I had no idea what that meant, but I was glad it was back as well. I suspected Julie was referring to the way I looked when we'd met 13 years earlier, but at that time I was fresh on the heels of a one-hundred-pound weight loss. Which, of course, would have made the "old Gary face" actually the "new Gary face" at the time. Is anybody following at this point? Hello 1-800 Tech support…

YOU KNOW YOU'RE ON YOUR WAY TO GETTING HEALTHY WHEN...

APRIL 2002

I walk past an obese guy walking the lake and nearly look down my nose at him in a *doesn't he have any respect for himself* type way. Luckily, I catch myself just in time to realize I was him just a year ago.

AUGUST 2002

I take my brother Rich to the Sam and Dave Tour (former Van Halen singers) at The Tweeter Center in Mansfield. During the show's last song, Sammy Hagar invites about 25 audience members, including my brother and myself, on stage for the show's big finale. I'm dancing center stage wearing my loudest Hawaiian shirt and not the least bit embarrassed or self-conscious of my weight. For a brief moment I'm even singing with Sammy in front of 8,000 people. A hundred pounds ago I wouldn't get up in front of a crowd in front of a Karaoke bar, and now I'm Elvis.

DECEMBER 2002

Sleep Apnea goes away—Merry Christmas!

JANUARY 2003

Julie and I spend the holidays in San Francisco, a town famous for its hills. I'm walking everywhere I go. No Rice-a-Roni train needed!

FEBRUARY 2003

Julie sautés fresh kale together with onions and rice vinegar to go with our weekly Sushi Dinner. I'm absolutely loving the kale dish. We're talking kale here, folks.

There I am complimenting my wife every 30 seconds on her tasty kale recipe as if it's some sort of lobster casserole. "Honey, I love this kale!," All of this from the guy who just two and a half years ago was spreading butter on his steaks.

MARCH 2003

As part of my Cardiac Risk Reduction class, I'm required to get an updated blood test performed. My doctor asks me to fast for 12 to 18 hours before the test. I'm not even the least bit phased. Two years ago the concept of fasting would have put me in therapy. Now I couldn't honestly care less.

APRIL 2003

Julie comes home from the supermarket with two orders of BBQ soy ribs for dinner. After I go through my usual routine of asking her why she would waste her time buying such a product for me, I try a bite. "Oh my God…that's great!" I blurt between bites. Then I proceed to eat both hers and mine. Delicious! Soy ribs. Who knew?

MAY 2003

I'm wearing my tee shirts on the inside out so that the tag sticks way out and people can see that I'm down to a size 1x. Well, at least someone's got his confidence back.

JUNE 2003

While working out at the gym I notice an attractive girl by the free weights wearing a spandex jumpsuit and a pair of weight-lifting gloves. It's not her long blond hair or sculptured body that hooks my attention; it's those tight-fitting weight-lifting gloves that I find so incredibly hot. I'm absolutely transfixed by the gloves she's wearing. Times, they are a-changing.

JULY 2003

The very first Krispy Crème Donut Shop holds its Massachusetts grand opening in none other but my hometown of Medford. It's a historic day. The Mayor is there. The media is there. Entire families are there. But a former 397 lb. food enthusiast who grew up just two miles away is *not* there.

AUGUST 2003

I order take-out food for Julie and me on the way home from work. The bag of takeout rides shotgun with me in the car. When I arrive home 20 minutes later, the bag is unopened and the food is untouched. My portion is eaten with my wife, much like a normal couple. Refreshing, huh?

SEPTEMBER 2003

In the gym locker room a fellow weight-lifter half jokingly tells me he needs to work out to burn off the hamburger he had for lunch. I respond by telling him to have a great workout. I ask no details whatsoever about the hamburger.

HALLOWEEN 2003

Before reluctantly handing out candy to trick-or-treaters, I consider having them sign legal waivers that read: "The Marino Family cannot be held accountable for the pediatric obesity epidemic currently gripping our neighborhood. "

DECEMBER 2003

I meet then-Democratic front-runner Howard Dean at a campaign event at the Park Plaza Hotel in Boston. During a conversation about the obesity issue, I inform Governor Dean that he has weapons of mass destruction in his home state of Vermont. "We do?" he asks alarmingly. "Yes; Ben & Jerry's," I respond "They're killing us!"

JANUARY 2004

At cocktail bars and lounges I talk to bartenders without wiping out the olives, cherries and other assorted items on their garnish trays.

TIME IS A TOOL

"These are better days, baby, better days are shining through…"

—*Bruce Springsteen*

It's getting easier. Consuming 1600 calories a day and eating healthier is actually getting easier. Why, after two and a half years, is it finally getting easier? Because one of the most important lessons an overweight person can learn is that time truly is a tool. In time, healthy foods will taste like a treat, just like junk foods used to. I know it's hard to believe, but trust me, it happens. It's a lesson that is essential for overcoming this disease. When I began back in 2000, meals like grilled chicken salads and broiled haddock with baby carrots did absolutely nothing for me. Eating them felt like a diet to me—like I was denying myself. In time (and we're only talking three to six months here), once I conditioned myself to eating these types of healthy meals, they were simply delicious to me. Over time I tweaked them by adding spices or dry-rub marinades. They became a way of life to me, and I actually felt good eating them, knowing they were in fact what my body needed. Even foods as simple as a cheeseburger changed with time. When I started, I was a cheeseburger addict. Give me two sub-par grade ground beef patties with melted cheddar, ketchup, mayonnaise, BBQ sauce and whatever, and I was in heaven. And hell hath no fury if they weren't between some kind of bulkie roll—onion, sesame seed, or the mother of all rolls: the Portuguese Sweet Bread Roll. Let's face it, you could put a slice of rubber in between Portuguese Sweet Bread and it would taste delicious. These days, I cook two four-ounce lean sirloin burgers on my George Forman grill with a slice of fat-free cheese, ketchup, grilled onions and a little ground pepper, and you'd think I was eating Filet Mignon from the way I oooh and aaaahh over it. I couldn't imagine wasting the flavor by bringing bread into the picture. Bread, as a matter of fact, had become a mere interruption to me. How can you enjoy the taste of your over-priced sirloin with bread firmly wrapped around it? I can't imagine. My point is that over time I turned cheeseburgers into a healthy meal and I love it as much as ever. Maybe even more so, because it's healthy. And I do not feel an ounce of denial. I swear.

When Melinda suggested I eat a small handful of raw almonds every day, I did not get excited. I had never been much of an almond or even nut guy. At first, eating them did nothing for me. I may as well have been taking a vitamin pill. I found them bland and unexciting. But in very short order I was an almond nut, popping them as a mid-morning snack and absolutely loving the flavor that did not seem to be there when I started.

Time is a tool, people, trust me. Low-calorie yogurt from the dairy section now tastes like Ben & Jerry's to me. Wheaties and a slice of banana in the morning are as delicious as Captain Crunch (Crunch Berries, to be specific) used to be. An Egg Beater omelet with a side of cottage cheese or applesauce does it for me just as did it's predecessor, a four-egg omelet with corned beef hash and American cheese. I just needed to seek these healthy foods out, accept that they were what my body truly needed, and give the process a little time. Any of the items I used to eat—the ones that wrecked my life for all those years—felt ridiculous and over-the-top to me. Melinda's words about not hating food but hating what my approach to it had done to my life rang true to me suddenly.

In time, even items like soda pop and orange juice seemed over-the-top to me. The soda was too sweet and provided my body with nothing, absolutely nothing. The juice thing is a yet another piece of nutrition that people, including myself, misunderstand. Healthy? Well, sort of. Too much sugar and fruit juice. One small glass and you've overdone all your fruits for the day. These days I drink water 98 percent of the time.

In time, even the slice of Americana known as the buffet became old hat to me. When I am at a buffet these days it feels like a warm bath of nostalgia to me. I revisit it. I appreciate it. I study the other patrons gorging themselves. I laugh at its ridiculousness. I pick out some healthy items or I treat myself, but then I move on. Food is fuel to me, not what life is all about.

Time is indeed a powerful tool, my friends. It can help you slowly change your destructive eating patterns. Motivational speaker Tony Robbins has a great book entitled *Awaken The Giant Within*. I guess what I'm talking about here is the polar opposite. Food addicts need to put the giant within into a sleep state. We need to let the unhealthy eating go and forget about the foods we grew up thinking were so good. They were, in my opinion, an aberration. If you can look at it this way, it's more than worth it, believe me. There's a great saying out there: "Nothing tastes as good as thin feels." Use time as your secret weapon and you'll appreciate it's truthfulness.

Here is a list of pointers I learned will work if you give them time:

1. If you are an anxiety eater like me, condition yourself to use fruit or vegetables as your emotional quick fix snack as opposed to Klondike Bars and Licorice.

2. Don't plan on taking a "treat day." The opportunity to treat yourself to the foods you love will present themselves naturally at least once a week. By not planning an actual day, you will be in good shape when a sudden dinner invitation happens or the pizza delivery guy mistakenly delivers that large extra cheese and pepperoni to your door.

3. By the same token, don't plan on taking a day off from exercising or working out to "let your muscles recover," as most trainers recommend. That opportunity, given today's hectic and pathetic schedules, will also present itself naturally. Exercise is always the easiest thing to get derailed on.

Time is not only a powerful tool for reconditioning your taste buds, but it is key to get you to the stage Melinda coined "Final Frontiers." I've written a lot about the process of dissecting in this book. In time you'll find yourself dissecting more than just what you put in your mouth. Eventually, you'll further dissect habits and patterns that are also unhealthy, such as sleeping routines, how you deal with anxiety, and finding serenity. These are very important final frontiers, because if you are an anxiety eater such as myself you'll need to cut down on your anxiety as much as possible. The "Final Frontiers" stage is about finding inner piece. With your food addiction and weight issues firmly under control and behind you you'll find the need to fine-tune other aspects of your life. As 280 pounds became 250, I found myself learning about things I used to dismiss as a crude joke. Yoga. Up until now the closest I'd ever gotten was yogurt. Now I'm beginning to understand its value. Meditation exercises, Pilates, and spiritual stuff are all key to ultimate happiness. Thanks to Melinda, all these things now make perfect sense to me. Nurturing your physical body is one type of health. Nurturing your mind and soul is truly another. Each is equally important, and for too many years I simply neglected both.

I was not alone. In America, we've all been accustomed to a certain style of eating. An abnormal style, but to us it's *normal*. Once we develop weight problems and go on a food plan that resembles anything that even remotely looks like a diet, we freak out about denying ourselves. The truth is, the food plan Melinda designed and customized for me is actually a healthy-way-of-life plan, not a diet in the customary "only until you lose the weight" sense. You'll get used to it. Trust me. MAD TV, the sketch comedy show on the Fox Network, used to spoof a dating service called "Lowered Expectations." I hate to say it, but lowered expectations are what we all need to have concerning how and what we consume. Food is fuel, not love. We need to get used to fruits and salads and healthy snacks and let go of the concept of gigantic portions, of "honey roasted" this or "butter whipped" that. We need to identify the legendary all-you-can-eat-buffet as good restaurant advertising but terrible nutrition. Most importantly, we need to understand that at some point, probably before we were born, the United States went far off course in its food production, farm subsidies, balanced nutrition, advertising, labeling, portion sizes and subsequent consumption. In the end, we will all pay the price. The fat, the skinny, the young and the folks lucky enough to live to be old. Even the millions of Americans who have never been affected by this disease will pay. As the obesity epidemic continues, their health care costs will soar. Many of their kids, their family, friends and loved ones will undoubtedly become overweight and suffer the consequences.

The good news is that in time, if we take responsibility for ourselves, look in the mirror, dissect our disorders, learn about nutrition, stop supporting the junk food manufacturers and incorporate exercise permanently into their lives, we *can* turn it around. Not in a year or two years, but maybe 10, 15 or 20. We can use time as a tool.

Time being a tool is the good news. The bad news? Eating healthy is expensive! But don't let the money part disrupt you; it's worth it!

My trainer Sharon once asked me what type of lettuce I was eating. "Umm, iceberg?" I answered, not exactly sure if my answer was the right one.

"You should eat Mesclun," Sharon responded.

"Wow, I haven't gone near that stuff since high school!" I joked.

"Mesclun lettuce," she retorted. "It's got the most vitamins of any lettuce. You should eat it," she suggested. Now like most folks, I thought lettuce was lettuce, but as I ventured deeper and deeper into the nutrition thing, the surprises kept coming. Later that day, while at the supermarket, I scouted the Mesclun lettuce. It actually looked healthier than the romaine and iceberg. It had reds and whites and greens, all in bite-sized pieces and almost designer shapes. I grabbed a plastic produce bag and began jamming the vitamin lettuce into the bag. Then, as the bag swelled, I caught a look at the price. $7.98 per pound. *Excuse me? Just what kind of vitamins are in this lettuce?* Next to it the romaine was advertised at $1.98 per pound. Initially, I began dumping the Mesclun back, eventually realizing two things. First, the stuff is light as a feather and a pound would last me a week. Second, that I would never, ever put a price on my health. If Mesclun lettuce was the healthiest, then I'd be overdosing on it. Amazing how I'd changed. Two years previously, my idea of health was a glass of orange juice between dinner courses. I went from the guy you couldn't approach about his weight to that guy blocking the supermarket aisle because he's comparing the nutritional facts.

As time went on, I began to eat a lot of fish. I'd try new recipes and incorporate them into my lifestyle. Now I love fish. Almond encrusted Haddock. I love it! Bluefish on the grill with low-carb, low-calorie Italian salad dressing? Give it to me 3 nights a week for all I care. The price may give you sticker shock as well. Two pounds of haddock at $6.99 per pound? $13.98. The old me wouldn't pay that, but these days I could care less. It's delicious and healthy, so bring it on.

Buying healthy foods was expensive, but not nearly as costly as staying fat. In the end, it was the same game it always had been. I just needed to have the desire. Exercise every day and eat healthy foods. And if you can afford it, go with the Mesclun.

GARY VERSION 2.0

If you can meet with triumph and disaster
And treat those two impostors just the same
If you can fill the unforgiving minute,
With 60 seconds worth of distance run
Yours is the earth and everything that's in it.
And—which is more—you'll be a Man, my Son!

—*Excerpt from "IF" by Rudyard Kipling*

I woke up in bed with Julie on a warm summer morning recently and felt a mass bulging underneath my skin at the bottom of my rib cage. *Cancer,* I thought. *This is it. The big one. Lose the weight and then lose your life. Just my luck.* Alarmed, I felt it again before waking my wife with the words that no significant other ever wants to hear. "Honey, feel this for a minute. I've got some sort of growth in my chest," I said. Julie looked concerned, even numb, as she reached over and placed her hand underneath where mine had been nervously groping for quite some time. A split second later an incredulous and ridiculous look came over her face. I believe it would qualify as a *you've got to be kidding me* look.

"That's your sternum. Oh my God, don't you know, that's your sternum?" She laughed.

"Is that a good thing?" I joked back.

Apparently, all the Cybex machines, free weights and cardio workouts had been having an effect after all. With a 130-pound obstacle removed, I now had a sternum at the base of my ribs.

Julie shook her head and rolled out of bed to put on coffee while I headed energetically for the bathroom mirror to see if could admire my recently uncovered sternum. But before I could obsess about it, something else caught my eye.

The face in the mirror. Somehow, it does not look the same. With each passing day it begins to look…healthy. One pound at a time and one workout at a time, the face that has greeted me each day for the better part of 15 years gradually disappears. Gone are the dark circles around my eyes, the strained puffy cheeks, and the uncomfortable look of an individual so very lost. And the chins! I'm down to one and a half, but give me time. The journey to health is truly a marathon, not a sprint.

People on the street walk past me these days and don't seem to recognize me. Heck, I don't even recognize myself half the time. Most mornings I actually do a double-take when I first look into the bathroom mirror. I'm…normal! Even energetic looking. The face that I now see each day has a few more lines on it, but it's the me I was meant to be at 38 years of age. The eyes have the look of a soldier whose battle for control is winding down. The disease has been defeated.

I left that morning to have breakfast with a friend. As I slowly poked away at my eggbeater omelet, fruit cup and cottage cheese, he marveled at my slow, methodical way of eating and my overall disinterest in the meal.

"Just an omelet? Aren't you going to order some sides?" my friend inquired. "Where are the home fries or your usual ice cream shakes? What's this? The new you?"

I stared at him confidently, and then responded with a smile. "You've got me confused with Gary Version 1.0," I said confidently. "This version is lighter, travels faster and handles even better." My, how things have changed. Just a few years earlier I would have asked for a scoop of vanilla ice cream in my coffee and a bed of corned beef hash to rest my cheese blintz on.

And that's not the only change here in the new era of Gary, Version 2.0. I'm actually finding myself excited and ready to become a father for the first time in my life. Perhaps it all coincides with my health goals being achieved. Maybe it's turning 38 years old. All I know is I woke up one day and there the feeling was. The days of delaying reality or second-guessing my physical capabilities are long gone. Are the 40s too old to start a family? Maybe for some people, but youth is a state of mind and body. From that perspective, I'm younger than I've been in 20 years. Call it "bucking the trend," but I've got more energy to change diapers and chase crawling babies than I ever had in my younger years. I'll be that father running around with his kid on his shoulders. The one sliding into first base. The one up early cooking breakfast—eggbeaters that is. And whether it's the sweetest of little girls or a little rebel like me, I promise they'll get plenty of love from their dad. I'll give them the things Rainbow gave to me. I'll make her proud, and like her, my kids will know that I'll never be too far away, even when I'm exploring other universes.

Not all that long ago, I walked the Mystic Lakes in West Medford near where our family grew up. As I always have, I stopped at Oak Grove Cemetery where Rainbow is buried. The sun was just beginning to fade behind the trees. I stood there for what seemed like hours, thinking about how proud she'd be of her son. I swear I could feel those amazing hazel green eyes smiling down on me from the heavens. In so many ways, she's really never left. This march towards health had always been about promises to keep: promises I made to my mother to get healthy and promises I made to myself about living life the way it was meant to be lived. It's been a long road, but in the end I believe I've come through on both counts. Something tells me life is going to be a lot sweeter this time around as a result.

Shortly after my mother's death, I began to feel as if this disease was given to me. We are all given our crosses to bear, and spiritually I believe my struggle in life was to overcome food addiction and get healthy. Losing weight, as most people know, is not simply a game of how much you lose, but rather how long you keep it off. With my ability to overeat now solidly under control, I feel I am truly ready to take on whatever else comes my way in life. Thinking back to the dark days of my Sleep Apnea and how resigned I was to the fact that I was dying, I now realize what a come-from-behind effort this has actually been. While I won't cry for yesterday, I'll always be in awe of the colossal effort and unique road it took to get me where I am.

Now, do I think everyone should start foundations, design cross-country walks and turn their daily journals into 300 pages of pure therapy? Of course not. No two people are the same, and everyone who seeks to get fit and healthy must find his or her own unique path to get there. It's out there for every one of us, if we're willing to find it.

As a person, I've always wanted to make an impact on this planet before I left. "Leave my mark," as you hear people say from time to time. Through the years, I always thought that mark would be as a musician, video producer, talent manager, actor, or a morning radio personality. You know, all the things people everywhere dream about doing everyday. However, if The Million Calorie March and the Generation Excel Foundation can inspire even one person to get healthy or light the fire under just a few of the countless people who have lost hope, then it's far more important than anything else I'd ever hoped to accomplish in my lifetime. And whether I'm able to inspire three people or 300,000, it's all the same spark, especially when we're talking about improving people's lives. When I began the bulk of this manuscript, 61 percent of Americans were overweight. As I near completion of this book, that statistic has grown to 65 percent. 100 people a week will die in Massachusetts alone as a result of the obesity epidemic, and one third of all children born in the year 2000 will develop type two diabetes. As long as the numbers continue like that, this recovered food addict isn't going anywhere. I'll stay and fight this epidemic long after I'm at my goal weight of 195 pounds.

Nationwide, despite obesity statistics getting worse, powerful changes are happening. We're beginning to see the start of a very real revolution out there these days. People in this country are beginning to question the foods they put into their bodies. They're starting to focus on how certain foods affect their physical and mental health. Every day, people are starting to dissect their eating patterns and understand themselves a little more. Most importantly, they are beginning to question how normal it was to eat so badly in the first place. Entire industries are beginning to recognize the coming changes as well.

Food manufactures like Kraft are redesigning their high-calorie, high-fat products such as Oreos for a more calorie conscious America. They are even pledging to make their serving sizes smaller and post their nutrition information on their labels worldwide. Soy products are popping up everywhere.

Some New York City schools are actually removing vending machines from their premises. In Boston, my old friend City Councilor John Tobin is leading an initiative to remove junk foods from the grammar schools and junior highs.

The FDA is stepping up to the plate and forcing food manufacturers to list transfats on their labels by 2006. McDonalds, the Uber fast food producers of the world, are actually doing away with their trademark super-sizing. Now if Ben &

Jerry's could actually take it down to half a dozen flavors, we'd become true believers! As for McDonalds, their new line of salads have sold so well it seems to have surprised even them, and their "Real Life" meals offer burgers without the buns. (I know, it sounds like a threat to me too!) Burger King is pushing its Chicken Whopper as if it's become their signature sandwich. Kentucky Fried Chicken (KFC) is now rebranding themselves "Kitchen Fresh Chicken." It seems that the majority of fast food companies are taking notice of the low carb craze and branding for a healthier society. Whether these corporations are concerned with their bottom lines or yours, the issue of true health is slowly beginning to etch its way into our nation's consciousness. Soon, the country's health experts may very well get the massive obesity prevention campaign they've been calling for. I, for one, will support it in any way I can.

Incidentally, as I write this, it appears that the Million Calorie March cross-country walk has found a second wind. Thanks to my friend and Harmon-Marino client Todd Patkin and a group of Boston businessmen who believe in my cause, money is being raised and the event seems to be picking up speed each day. Who knows? Maybe I was actually on to something back in early 2001. If I was, I'll be seeing you down the road very soon. In the meantime, if you are caught in the weight loss struggle, face it head on. Don't be discouraged if it takes a long time to achieve your goals. Complex problems take time to fix! I promise you will never hear me boast that I lost the weight in 20 years flat. Most importantly, do not, under any circumstances, accept your predicament as a fact of life.

In the end, I hope that chronicling all of these *MisAdventures* serves a greater purpose than just aiding the folks dealing with weight problems. I hope that this book gives the many people who have never experienced eating disorders some valuable insight into the lives of people who do. I hope it helps you to size up what's in their souls first and foremost, before anything else. Remember, they feel worse on the inside than they ever could look like on the outside.

As you know, "The Million Calorie March" is more than a cross-country weight loss walk; it's a metaphor for my journey to health. Now it may seem as if this *March* was a one-man quest, but the truth is, I could never have completed it without the help of the very best people on Earth. My body may have become smaller throughout this experience, but as my brother Richard says, I'm now a "fit guy with an obese heart." I am forever indebted to the people who helped me accomplish my victory over the control of this disease. They have truly given me a second chance at life.

To my wife Julie, my family, co-workers, clients and friends who never stopped supporting me through my entire journey to health, thank you all from the bottom of my heart. To the corporations, activists and well-meaning folks who continue to get involved with the Generation Excel Project to help improve the quality of people's lives everywhere, I'm forever grateful. Finally, to the Dream Team of Melinda Vaturro, Ruth Schwartz, Vincent Zarella, Sharon Cummings and Dr. Bertram Zarens, thank you! Thanks for making this chubby Italian boy's dreams become a reality.

As a result of these amazing people, my Million Calorie March experience has been the absolute ride of a lifetime. I'm humbled and—well, winded. It may sound cliché, but this book has been a very long way of saying that if I can beat this disease, anyone can. And you can. Continue to focus on your health. Dissect your disorders. Analyze your eating habits. Face your truths so you can watch the miracles happen. And most of all, when it comes to your dreams, head straight towards them and keep on *marching*.

The End...
or
The Beginning

ABOUT THE AUTHOR

Gary Marino began writing in the late 1980s as a radio producer in Boston. For the past ten years he has owned and operated Harmon-Marino Entertainment, where in addition to producing television pilots, live shows and videos, he writes scripts, treatments and comedy monologues.

In 2004, he launched The Million Calorie March, a first-of-its-kind 1,200-mile weight loss walk up the east coast, which reached over 70 million people. He is also the founder of Generation Excel, a nonprofit foundation dedicated to fighting obesity in children and adults by funding and promoting nutrition and physical fitness programs. *Big & Tall Chronicles* is his first book.

For more information, visit www.millioncaloriemarch.com

0-595-32154-2